Use of Sonography in Upper Extremity Surgery: Innovative Concepts and Techniques

Editors

FRÉDÉRIC A. SCHUIND
FABIAN MOUNGONDO
LUC VAN OVERSTRAETEN

HAND CLINICS

www.hand.theclinics.com

Consulting Editor
KEVIN C. CHUNG

February 2022 • Volume 38 • Number 1

ELSEVIER

1600 John F. Kennedy Boulevard • Suite 1800 • Philadelphia, Pennsylvania, 19103-2899

http://www.theclinics.com

HAND CLINICS Volume 38, Number 1
February 2022 ISSN 0749-0712, ISBN-13: 978-0-323-83578-7

Editor: Lauren Boyle
Developmental Editor: Hannah Almira Lopez

Hand Clinics (ISSN 0749-0712) is published quarterly by Elsevier Inc., 360 Park Avenue South, New York, NY 10010-1710. Months of publication are February, May, August, and November. Business and Editorial Offices: 1600 John F. Kennedy Blvd., Ste. 1800, Philadelphia, PA 19103-2899. Customer Service Office: 3251 Riverport Lane, Maryland Heights, MO 63043. Periodicals postage paid at New York, NY and at additional mailing offices. Subscription price is $444.00 per year (domestic individuals), $1060.00 per year (domestic institutions), $100.00 per year (domestic students/residents), $506.00 per year (Canadian individuals), $1081.00 per year (Canadian institutions), $568.00 per year (international individuals), $1081.00 per year (international institutions), $256.00 (international students/residents), and $100.00 (Canadian students/residents). Foreign air speed delivery is included in all *Clinics* subscription prices. All prices are subject to change without notice. **POSTMASTER:** Send address changes to *Hand Clinics*, Elsevier Health Sciences Division, Subscription Customer Service, 3251 Riverport Lane, Maryland Heights, MO 63043. Customer Service (orders, claims, online, change of address): Elsevier Health Sciences Division, Subscription **Customer Service, 3251 Riverport Lane, Maryland Heights, MO 63043. Tel: 1-800-654-2452 (U.S. and Canada); 314-447-8871 (outside U.S. and Canada). Fax: 314-447-8029. E-mail: journalscustomerservice-usa@elsevier.com (for print support); journalsonlinesupport-usa@elsevier.com (for online support)**.

Reprints. For copies of 100 or more of articles in this publication, please contact the Commercial Reprints Department, Elsevier Inc., 360 Park Avenue South, New York, New York 10010-1710. Tel.: 212-633-3874; Fax: 212-633-3820; E-mail: reprints@elsevier.com.

Hand Clinics is covered in *MEDLINE/PubMed (Index Medicus), Current Contents/Clinical Medicine, EMBASE/Excerpta Medica,* and *ISI/BIOMED.*

Contributors

CONSULTING EDITOR

KEVIN C. CHUNG, MD, MS
Charles B.G. de Nancrede Professor of
Surgery, Professor of Plastic Surgery and
Orthopaedic Surgery, Chief of Hand Surgery,
Michigan Medicine, Assistant Dean for Faculty
Affairs, Associate Director of Global REACH,
University of Michigan Medical School, Ann
Arbor, Michigan, USA

EDITORS

FRÉDÉRIC A. SCHUIND, MD, PhD
Department of Orthopaedics and
Traumatology, Erasme University Hospital,
Brussels, Belgium

FABIAN MOUNGONDO, MD, PhD
Department of Orthopaedics and
Traumatology, ULB Erasme University

Hospital, Université Libre de Bruxelles,
Brussels, Belgium

LUC VAN OVERSTRAETEN, MD, PhD
Department of Orthopaedics and
Traumatology, Erasme University Hospital,
Brussels, Belgium; Hand and Wrist Center,
HFSU, AO Foundation, Tournai, Belgium

AUTHORS

AMR MOHAMED ALY, MD
Associate Professor, Department of
Orthopaedics, Ain Shams University Hospital,
Cairo, Egypt

KAI-NAN AN, PhD
Professor Emeritus, Mayo Clinic College of
Medicine, Rochester, Minnesota, USA

THOMAS APARD, MD, FEBHS
Ultrasound Hand Surgery Center, Versailles,
France

FRANÇOIS BAUZOU, MD
Service de Chirurgie Orthopedique et
Traumatologique, Centre Hospitalo-
Universitaire Caremeau, Nimes, France

STEFANO BIANCHI, MD
CIM SA, Cabinet d'imagerie médicale, Geneva,
Switzerland

EMMANUEL JACQUES CAMUS, MD, PhD
Department of Orthopaedic and Traumatologic
Surgery, University Clinical Center, Polyclinic
Val de Sambre, Maubeuge, France

TAI-CHANG CHERN, MD
Tai-Chung Chern's Orthopedics Clinic, Ping-
Tung, Taiwan

SAMUEL CHRISTEN, MD
Hand, Plastic and Reconstructive Surgery,
Cantonal Hospital St. Gallen, St Gallen,
Switzerland

JEAN MICHEL COGNET, MD
SOS Mains Champagne Ardenne, Médipôle,
Bezannes, France

VIVIANE CRÉTEUR, MD
Department of Radiology, CUB Hôpital
Erasme, Université Libre de Bruxelles,
Brussels, Belgium

ISABELLE DAVID, MD
Department of Hand Surgery, Belledonne Private Hospital, Saint-Martin d'Hères, France

VÉRONIQUE FEIPEL, MD, PhD
Laboratory of Functional Anatomy, Faculty of Motor Sciences, Université Libre de Bruxelles, Brussels, Belgium

HUGO GIAMBINI, PhD
Assistant Professor, Department of Biomedical Engineering and Chemical Engineering, The University of Texas at San Antonio, College of Engineering and Integrated Design, San Antonio, Texas, USA

YOSHIFUMI HARADA, PhD, MD
Department of Orthopaedic Surgery, Kobe Rosai Hospital, Kobe, Japan

ATSUYUKI INUI, PhD, MD
Department of Orthopaedic Surgery, Kobe University Graduate School of Medicine, Kobe, Japan

I-MING JOU, MD, PhD
Department of Orthopedics, E-Da Hospital, School of Medicine, College of Medicine, I-Shou University, Kaohsiung, Taiwan

TAKAKO KANATANI, PhD, MD
Department of Orthopaedic Surgery, Kobe Rosai Hospital, Kobe, Japan

RONNY KINANGA, MD
Department of Orthopaedics and Traumatology, Erasme University Hospital, Université libre de Bruxelles, Brussels, Belgium

SEBASTIAN KLUGE, MD
Handchirurgie Seefeld, Zurich, Switzerland; Department of Hand Surgery, Klinik Impuls, Wetzikon, Switzerland

LI-CHIEH KUO, PhD
Medical Device Innovation Center, National Cheng Kung University, Department of Occupational Therapy, College of Medicine, National Cheng Kung University, Tainan, Taiwan

RYOSUKE KURODA, PhD, MD
Department of Orthopaedic Surgery, Kobe University Graduate School of Medicine, Kobe, Japan

MARTIN LANGER, MD
Department of Trauma, Hand and Reconstructive Surgery, University of Munster, Munster, Germany

PASCAL LOUIS, MD
SOS Mains Champagne Ardenne, Medipole, Bezannes, France

AFARINE MADANI, MD, PhD
Service de Radiologie, Department of Radiology, CUB Hôpital Erasme, Université Libre de Bruxelles, Brussels, Belgium

OLIVIER MARES, MD
Service de Chirurgie Orthopédique et Traumatologique, Centre Hospitalo-Universitaire Carémeau, Nîmes, France

YUTAKA MIFUNE, PhD, MD
Department of Orthopaedic Surgery, Kobe University Graduate School of Medicine, Kobe, Japan

FABIAN MOUNGONDO, MD, PhD
Department of Orthopaedics and Traumatology, ULB Erasme University Hospital, Université Libre de Bruxelles, Brussels, Belgium

ISSEI NAGURA, PhD, MD
Department of Orthopedic Surgery, Ako City Hospital, Ako, Japan

THOMAS SCHELLE, MD
Department of Neurology, Klinikum Dessau-Rosslau, Dessau-Rosslau, Germany

FRÉDÉRIC A. SCHUIND, MD, PhD
Department of Orthopaedics and Traumatology, Erasme University Hospital, Brussels, Belgium

CHUNG-JUNG SHAO, MD
Department of Orthopedics, Tainan Municipal Hospital, Tainan, Taiwan

FUMIAKI TAKASE, PhD, MD
Department of Orthopaedic Surgery, Kobe Rosai Hospital, Kobe, Japan

ESTHER VÖGELIN, MD
Professor, Hand Surgery and Surgery of Peripheral Nerves, Plastic and Hand Surgery Inselspital, University Hospital of Bern, Bern, Switzerland

LUC VAN OVERSTRAETEN, MD, PhD
Department of Orthopaedics and
Traumatology, Erasme University Hospital,
Brussels, Belgium; Hand and Wrist
Center, HFSU, AO Foundation, Tournai,
Belgium

KUO-CHEN WU, MD
Department of Orthopedics, Kuo's General
Hospital, Tainan, Taiwan

PO-TING WU, MD, PhD
Department of Orthopedics, College of
Medicine, Department of Biomedical
Engineering, Medical Device Innovation
Center, National Cheng Kung University,
Department of Orthopedics, National Cheng
Kung University Hospital, Tainan, Taiwan

TUNG-TAI WU, MD, PhD
GEG Orthopedics Clinic, Tainan, Taiwan

Contents

Accurate knowledge of the technique of ultrasonographic (US) examination and of normal US appearance is a prerequisite for a successful US examination of the wrist and hand. In this article, we describe our standard US examination as well as the normal US findings of the hand and wrist.

 Video content accompanies this article at http://www.hand.theclinics.com.

Ultrasonography in hand surgery offers the option of imaging trauma consequences or degenerative problems in the wrist and fingers, involving bones, joints, ligaments, tendons, annular pulley, carpal and digital changes, soft masses, and foreign bodies including dynamic changes during motion. In the hands of the treating surgeon, ultrasonography allows immediately to plan conservative treatment versus surgery, to precisely infiltrate joints or tendon spaces as well as to perform miniinvasive assisted surgery.

 Video content accompanies this article at http://www.hand.theclinics.com.

Ultrasonography is the best examination to explore the flexor tendons anatomy and disorders from the wrist to the digit. It is the only dynamic and comparative tool easily accessible for the surgeon. Indeed, ultrasonography is always available in all the departments of your hospital. Recent innovations permit to see superficially (high-frequency probes), precisely (smaller probes), and with greater softwares for an effective Doppler mode. Ultrasonography becomes a very important help at the outpatient clinic examination. In the future it can be used in the operating room to perform miniinvasive surgery under local anesthesia to control active motion of the gliding of flexor tendons.

 Video content accompanies this article at http://www.hand.theclinics.com.

Diagnostic ultrasound in the diagnosis of carpal tunnel syndrome is firmly established. Preoperative evaluation is based on quantitative parameters such as measurement of the pathologically enlarged cross-sectional area of the nerve. The value of postoperative ultrasound lies in the visualization of the anatomy and the conclusions that can be drawn from it. It focuses on the semiquantitative sonographic parameters of nerve compression. Nerve lesions and persistent strictures can be visualized and clearly localized. In recurrent disease, the primary focus is to dynamically exclude postoperative scarring, which results in a reduction of nerve gliding.

This article aims to evaluate the usefulness of ultrasonography for the measurement of thenar muscles in carpal tunnel syndrome (CTS). A total of 85 patients with CTS who had a carpal tunnel release procedure were included in this study. The transducer was applied onto the palmar surface of the hand perpendicularly to the longitudinal axis of the first metacarpal bone. Thenar atrophy was evaluated visually and classified using the visual grading scale. A nerve conduction test was performed and classified according to the electrophysiological severity scale. This technique is more precise than visual evaluation because it is a quantitative assessment.

Short procedures constitute a large proportion of hand surgeries. Most of them are done as 1-day surgery. Regional anesthesia is considered the best option for these operations. Compared with general anesthesia, regional anesthesia improves early outcome after wrist and hand surgery. Distal nerve blocks have the benefits of lying away from critical structures and the preservation of proximal muscle function of the upper limb. Thus, this type of nerve block is ideal for short procedures where patients can tolerate a tourniquet.

Percutaneous carpal tunnel release (CTR) is a new surgical technique allowing to cut the transverse carpal ligament under sonography, without skin incision. The technique is safe, offers good functional results and early return to daily activities. This study investigates if percutaneous CTR is also cost-effective. Percutaneous CTR presents many advantages and may be safer than open and endoscopic CTR. This study could not demonstrate that it allows also cheaper surgery, at least as compared to open CTR. However, if it allows earlier return to work, percutaneous CTR could offer a major economic advantage over other techniques, particularly open surgery.

 Video content accompanies this article at http://www.hand.theclinics.com.

During the past 2 decades, increased powerful and quality ultrasound devices have contributed to developing ultrasound surgery more specifically for the hand. Carpal tunnel release under ultrasound now is available as a safe technique. The procedure uses a specific device. A detailed surgical technique is presented. The role of sonography is emphasized. This article discusses the results of the 150 first cases. The author's experience is compared with other ultrasound-guided carpal tunnel release procedures. Outcome quality optimized by the ultra–mini-invasive approach and ultrasound should increase its use.

Safe Zones for Percutaneous Carpal Tunnel Release   83

Po-Ting Wu, Tai-Chang Chern, Tung-Tai Wu, Chung-Jung Shao, Kuo-Chen Wu, Li-Chieh Kuo, and I-Ming Jou

Carpal tunnel release (CTR) is an effective procedure used in open, endoscopic, or ultrasound-guided methods. The complications are rare but potentially devasting. Most complications come from errors related to intraoperative technique, especially in the minimally invasive approach. An understanding of the "safe zones" is essential to perform percutaneous CTR safely. This article reviews the anatomy of safe zones and the ultrasound-guided CTR (UCTR) techniques in an attempt to prevent intraoperative complications. In strict accordance with the concepts of safe zones, UCTR is an effective and reliable procedure. Substantial experience for ultrasound-guided injection and surgery is required.

Percutaneous Sonographically Guided Release of Carpal Tunnel and Trigger Finger: Biomechanics, Clinical Results, Technical Developments   91

Fabian Moungondo and Véronique Feipel

 Video content accompanies this article at http://www.hand.theclinics.com.

The interventional use of sonography is growing fast, and percutaneous sonographically guided release is more and more used as minimally invasive treatment of carpal tunnel syndrome as well as trigger finger digit. The benefits of these procedures seem promising in clinical studies, but biomechanical studies comparing these procedures with open classical surgery are scarce. Minimally invasive releases of carpal tunnel and trigger finger could limit the phenomenon of tendon bowstringing observed after open surgery. A new model is presented to compare the biomechanical effects of open and sono-guided carpal tunnel and trigger finger releases.

Volar Ganglion Cyst and Echo-Guided Assistance for the Arthroscopic Removal   101

Luc Van Overstraeten, Emmanuel Jacques Camus, Fabian Moungondo, and Frédéric Schuind

 Video content accompanies this article at http://www.hand.theclinics.com.

The ganglion of the wrist is very common but with uncertain prognosis. The arthroscopic resection seems to improve the result compared with open procedure, in decreasing recurrence and morbidity. Volar ganglions are close to the radial artery, the flexor pollicis longus tendon, and even the median nerve. Ultrasonography combined with arthroscopy offers incomparable safety for the resection of volar ganglions. The technical steps of this combined procedure are described, and the first published series are discussed.

Contents

Ultrasonography (US) is a noninvasive examination modality that is devoid of risk, both for the patient and the surgeon, compared with fluoroscopy. The principle is the same for distal radius and finger fractures: replace the fluoroscopy checks with US checks to reduce the patient's, surgeon's, and surgical team's exposure to radiation. In this article, the authors report their experience of the effectiveness of ultrasound imaging during the fixation of a distal radius and long finger fracture. They also describe equipment needed and surgical procedure.

Over the past decade, ultrasound elastography has emerged as a new technique for measuring soft tissue properties. Real-time, noninvasive, and quantitative evaluations of tissue stiffness have improved and aid in the assessment of normal and pathological conditions. Specifically, its use has substantially increased in the evaluation of muscle, tendon, and ligament properties. In this review, the authors describe the principles of elastography and present different techniques including strain elastography and shear-wave elastography; discuss their applications for assessing soft tissues in the hand before, during, and postsurgeries; present the strengths and limitations of their measurement capabilities; and describe directions for future research.

HAND CLINICS

SERIES OF RELATED INTEREST:

Clinics in Plastic Surgery
https://www.plasticsurgery.theclinics.com/

Orthopedic Clinics of North America
https://www.orthopedic.theclinics.com/

Physical Medicine and Rehabilitation Clinics of North America
https://www.pmr.theclinics.com/

THE CLINICS ARE AVAILABLE ONLINE!
Access your subscription at:
www.theclinics.com

HAND CLINICS

Preface

Use of Sonography in Hand/ Upper-Extremity Surgery: Innovative Concepts and Techniques

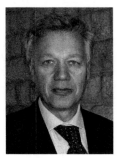

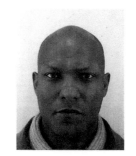

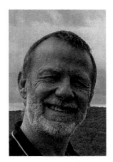

Frédéric A. Schuind, MD, PhD   Fabian Moungondo, MD, PhD   Luc Van Overstraeten, MD, PhD

Editors

Upper-extremity and hand surgeons are disposed nowadays of a new tool for diagnosis and to guide their operations: sonography. The recent improvements of this imaging modality allow excellent visualization of hand anatomic structures. Sonography has been proven invaluable in the outpatient clinic, to immediately confirm a suspicion of tendon rupture, to assess tendon gliding, to understand the nature of a hand tumor, and to confirm a suspected diagnosis of carpal tunnel syndrome or of scapholunate ligament tear, to give a few examples. In the outpatient clinic, sonography is now to the hand surgeon as the stethoscope is to the cardiologist. With the use of sterile gel and a cover for the probes, sonography now goes to into the operating room and helps for exposure and minimally invasive repair. It can be combined to electrostimulate nerves, for C-arm imaging, or for arthroscopy. Sonography can "simply" be used to guide a difficult dissection of fibrotic tissue, to preserve important neurovascular structures. In peripheral nerve surgery, sonography allows perioperative assessment of nerve dynamics and fascicular structure. Sonography can also help in the reduction of hand and wrist fractures. The most promising use of sonography is to guide minimally invasive release of trigger finger, carpal tunnel, de Quervain, and lateral epicondylitis and to perform percutaneous fasciotomy in Dupuytren and even percutaneous tenolysis. Indeed, the new surgical sonography-guided possibilities seem endless. Much remains to be developed, and the potential benefits and risks of the new procedures need to be carefully assessed.

The 28th Brussels/Genval Hand/Upper Limb Symposium had for their topic, "Perioperative Use of Sonography in Hand/Upper-Extremity Surgery—Innovative Concepts and Techniques," and should have taken place in Belgium in March 2020. The Congress had to be delayed, given the current COVID-19 pandemic, and is still on hold, waiting for an improvement in the situation. This issue of *Hand Clinics* includes several presentations that could not be given in Genval, in addition to other

Hand Clin 38 (2022) xiii–xiv
https://doi.org/10.1016/j.hcl.2021.08.014
0749-0712/22/© 2021 Published by Elsevier Inc.

contributions of invited colleagues experienced in hand sonography.

Frédéric A. Schuind, MD, PhD
Department of Orthopaedics and Traumatology
Erasme University Hospital
808 route de Lennik
Brussels, Belgium

Fabian Moungondo, MD, PhD
Orthopaedics and Traumatology
ULB Erasme Hospital
Brussels, Belgium

Luc Van Overstraeten, MD, PhD
Department of Orthopaedics and Traumatology
Erasme University Hospital
Brussels, Belgium

Hand and Wrist Center, HFSU
AO Foundation
Tournai, Belgium

E-mail addresses:
Frederic.Schuind@erasme.ulb.ac.be
(F.A. Schuind)
Fabian.Moungondo@erasme.ulb.ac.be
(F. Moungondo)
Luc.van.overstraeten@skynet.be (L. Van Overstraeten)

Atlas of Sonographic Anatomy of the Hand and Wrist

Afarine Madani, MD, PhD[a], Viviane Créteur, MD[b],*, Stefano Bianchi, MD[c]

KEYWORDS

- US • Hand • Wrist • Atlas • Normal anatomy

KEY POINTS

- Understanding US indications.
- Understanding US technique.
- Learning normal US appearance of wrist, hand, and fingers.

INTRODUCTION

X-rays have been traditionally used for the evaluation of bones, joints, and soft tissue calcifications.[1] In recent years, the role of musculoskeletal ultrasonography (US), particularly in the wrist and hand, has expanded dramatically for both diagnostic and interventional purposes.[2–4] Three main conditions are essential to perform an optimal US examination of the wrist and hand.

The first condition is equipment quality and standardized examination technique. Optimal equipment includes high-frequency linear array transducers ranging from 10 to 15 MHz, with an adapted size and shape of the probe, like a hockey-stick probe; Doppler imaging; compound imaging; extended field-of-view imaging; steering-based imaging; 3-dimensional imaging; elastography; contrast media; and DICOM capacities for static and dynamic recording.[5] Standardization of US examination technique involves examination first on the short axis and then on the long axis plane, performing dynamic evaluation, and correct focusing.

The second condition is appropriate US indications, pertinent clinical information, and patient's history.

The third condition is accurate interpretation of the images and correlation of the US findings with clinical data.

US may be applied to the bone as an adjunct to x-rays in selected cases because it can detect superficial cortical outgrowths or ingrowths.[6–9]

The US appearance of muscles and tendons is well known.[10,11] Normal skeletal muscles appear relatively hypoechoic with hyperechoic linear strands or dots, whereas normal tendons and ligaments appear highly hyperechoic because of their tight and compact fibrillar pattern. Tendons, like ligaments, are subject to anisotropy.[12,13]

In transverse view, nerves appear as round/ovoid structures composed of hypoechoic spots, corresponding to fascicles, embedded in a hyperechoic background, corresponding to the interfascicular epineurium.[11] In longitudinal view, they appear as fascicular structures composed of hypoechoic parallel linear areas separated by hyperechoic bands.[14,15]

[a] Service de Radiologie, Department of Radiology, CUB Hôpital Erasme, Université Libre de Bruxelles, 808, Route de Lennik, Brussels 1070, Belgium; [b] Department of Radiology, CUB Hôpital Erasme, Université Libre de Bruxelles, 808, Route de Lennik, Brussels 1070, Belgium; [c] CIM SA, Cabinet d'imagerie médicale, 40a route de Malagnou, Geneva 1208, Switzerland
* Corresponding author. 40, rue Haut du village, Sautour 5600, Belgium.
E-mail address: viviane.creteur@gmail.com

Hand Clin 38 (2022) 1–17
https://doi.org/10.1016/j.hcl.2021.08.001

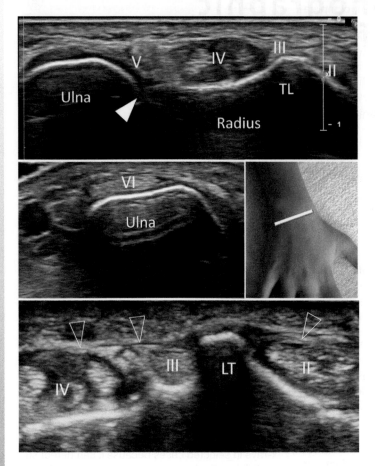

Fig. 1. At the dorsal wrist, 3 key structures are noticeable on an axial view: the dorsal tubercle of the radius, the extensor retinaculum (*open arrowheads*), and the distal radioulnar joint (*arrowhead*). The extensor retinaculum divides the dorsal wrist into 6 distinct compartments (I–VI). LT, lunotriquetral ligament; TL, Lister tubercle.

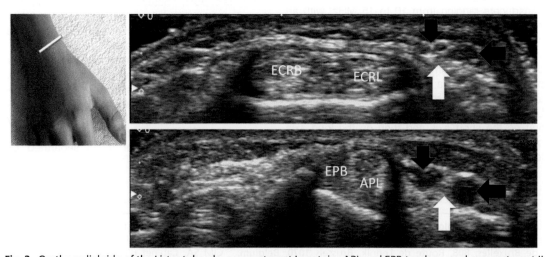

Fig. 2. On the radial side of the Lister tubercle, compartment I contains APL and EPB tendons, and compartment II contains ECRB and ECRL tendons. The cutaneous branch of the radial nerve (*white arrows*) and the cephalic vein (*black arrows*) are visible near these tendons. Excessive pressure of the probe may avoid visualization of small structures, such as superficial veins and nerves. APL, abductor pollicis longus; ECRB, extensor carpi radialis brevis; ECRL, extensor carpi radialis longus; EPB, extensor pollicis brevis.

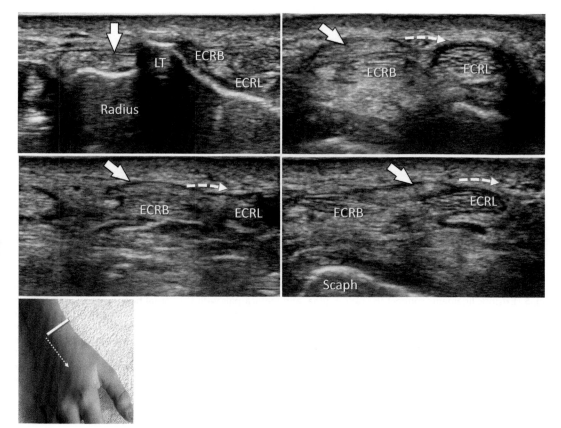

Fig. 3. When using the "elevator technique" from the Lister tubercle toward the scaphoid bone, axial US images display the proximal intersection of the radial tendons. The EPL tendon (compartment III, *white arrow*) crosses (*dotted curved arrow*) the ECRB and ECRL tendons (compartment II). This peculiar anatomic situation may lead to the so-called intersection syndrome, which is usually secondary to occupational repetitive flexion and extension of the wrist. This condition may be easily confused with De Quervain disease.Dotted arrow on artwork illustrates the axial progression of the probe from proximal to distal wrist. EPL, extensor pollicis longus; ECRB, extensor carpi radialis brevis; ECRL, extensor carpi radialis longus; Scaph, scaphoid.

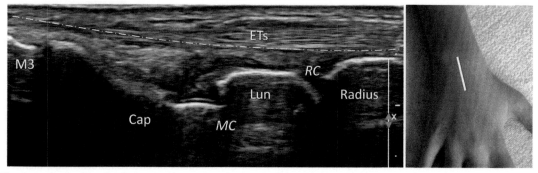

Fig. 4. In the longitudinal view performed at the level of the third metacarpal, carpal bone outlines are hyperechoic, regular, and relatively straight (*straight dotted line*). The RC and MC joints are visible. This view allows quick detection of synovial thickening or fluid. Cap, capitate; ETs, extensor tendons; Lun, lunate; MC, midcarpal joint; RC, radiocarpal joint.

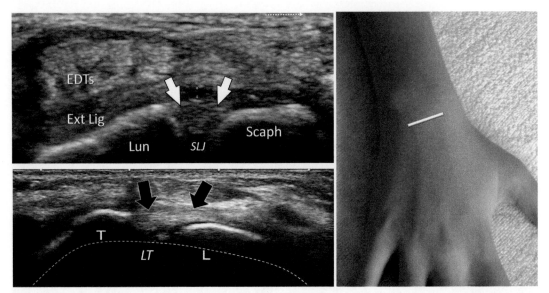

Fig. 5. Extrinsic ligaments connect the radius, ulna, and metacarpals with the carpal bones. These ligaments are partially visible underneath the extensor digitorum tendons, close to the bones. Intrinsic ligaments connect the carpal bones to one another. The most relevant ligaments seen on US are the SL (*white arrows*) and LT (*black arrows*) ligaments. These ligaments are better visualized on axial views. Observe that the carpal bones appear convex (*curved dotted line*) in the dorsal axial view but concave in the palmar axial view (see carpal tunnel, **Fig. 13**). EDTs, extensor digitorum communis tendons; Ext Lig, extrinsic ligament; L, Lu, lunate; SL, scapholunate ligament; SLJ, scapholunate joint; T, triquetrum.

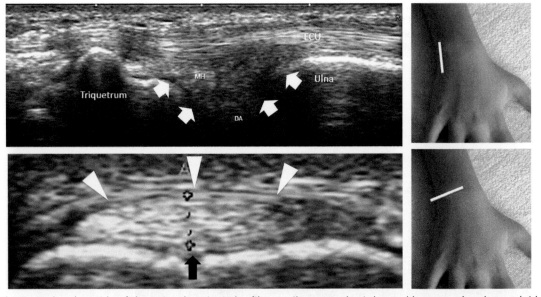

Fig. 6. At the ulnar side of the wrist, the triangular fibrocartilage complex is located between the ulnar styloid and distal radius (white arrows). The complex is composed of the triangular biconcave fibrocartilage, meniscus homologue, ulnar collateral ligament, radioulnar ligaments, and sheath (*arrowheads*) of the ECU (*black arrow*). Even with high-resolution transducers, US cannot distinguish the different components of the triangular fibrocartilage complex. Their accurate evaluation requires other modalities such as MRI or computed tomography with arthrography. DA, deep arterial arch; ECU, extensor carpi ulnaris; MH, meniscus homologue.

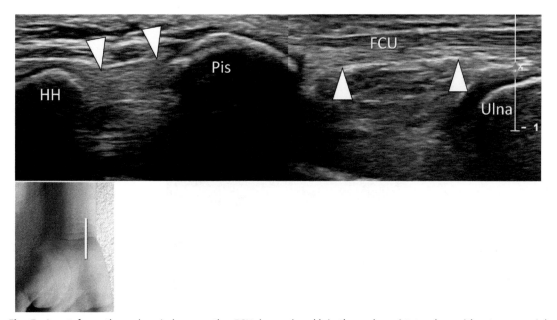

Fig. 7. Apart from the palmaris longus, the FCU (*arrowheads*) is the only wrist tendon without a synovial sheath. The FCU inserts into the pisiform. The pisohamate ligament is a prolongation of the FCU and serves as part of the origin of the ADM. ADM, adductor digiti minimi; FCU, flexor carpi ulnaris; HH, hamate hook; Pis, pisiform.

The US appearance of normal vessels has been documented. Compared with arteries, veins have thinner walls and larger lumens. In the wrist and hand, these vessels are relatively superficial, and their location may be easier to detect with color Doppler US.[16]

In this practical pictorial, we review the essentials of the US anatomy of the wrist and the hand.

Anatomic Structures Detected on Ultrasonography

Wrist: carpal joints, selected ligaments (scapholunate, lunotriquetral, and pisohamate ligaments), flexor and extensor tendons, retinacula, and neurovascular structures.[2–4,16]

Hand: muscles, joints, several ligaments (collateral metacarpophalangeal ligament of the thumb, collateral radial metacarpophalangeal ligament of the index, collateral ulnar metacarpophalangeal ligament of the fifth finger, and interphalangeal collateral ligaments), palmar plate, flexor and extensor tendons, palmar aponeurosis, annular pulleys, and neurovascular structures.[17–21]

Normal Ultrasonographic Anatomy of the Wrist and Hand

Although the position of the wrist and hand, as well as the location of the sonographer, may differ in the operating room of the surgeon than in the consultant room of the radiologist, the realization of US must be similar: beginning with axial views using the "elevator technique" and anatomic landmarks and followed by longitudinal images. Then, US images are obtained in different positions of the wrist and hand (such as flexion, extension, radial and ulnar deviation, pronation, supination, and active and passive movements), allowing dynamic evaluation of the region. US assessment of the wrist and hand should be complete, although extra attention could be paid to a special finding or a particular region of clinical interest.

To facilitate the interpretation of typical US images, the extensor (dorsal) and flexor (palmar) regions must be considered separately. Typically, the wrist must be examined first in the axial and longitudinal planes (dorsal followed by volar aspects), and then each finger must be examined

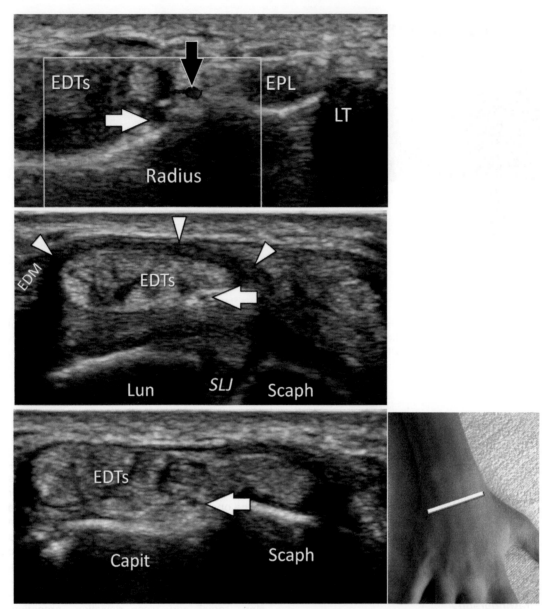

Fig. 8. At the ulnar side of the Lister tubercle, compartments III–V contain the EPL, EDTs, and EDM, respectively. The extensor retinaculum (*arrowheads*) surrounding the extensor tendons is clearly identified. The posterior interosseous nerve (*white arrow*) is deeply located and is accompanied by its artery (*black arrow*), which is easily identified using color Doppler US. This small nerve innervates only the dorsal wrist capsule and intra-articular structures. EDM, extensor digiti minimi; Capit, Capitate.

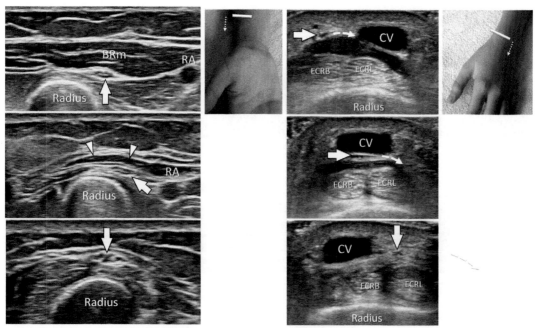

Fig. 9. The radial artery courses superficially with the radial nerve (*white arrow*) over the volar aspect of the distal radius, deep to the BRm and its tendon (*arrowheads*). The radial nerve then curves dorsally over the dorsal aspect of the wrist. At the distal radial aspect of the forearm, the superficial cutaneous branch of the radial nerve reaches the subcutaneous tissue between the ECRL and ECRB tendons, close to the cephalic vein (*curved dotted arrow*). BRm, brachioradialis muscle; CV, cephalic vein; RA, radial artery.

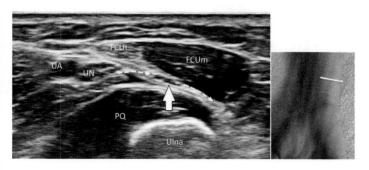

Fig. 10. In the distal volar forearm, the UN is located between the radial side of the FCUt and FCUm and the ulnar side of the UA. The UN gives off the dorsal cutaneous branch (*white arrow*) that runs between the FCUm superficially and the PQ deeply (*curved dotted arrow*). FCUm, flexor carpi ulnaris muscle; FCUt, flexor carpi ulnaris tendon; PQ, pronator quadratus; UA, ulnar artery; UN, ulnar nerve.

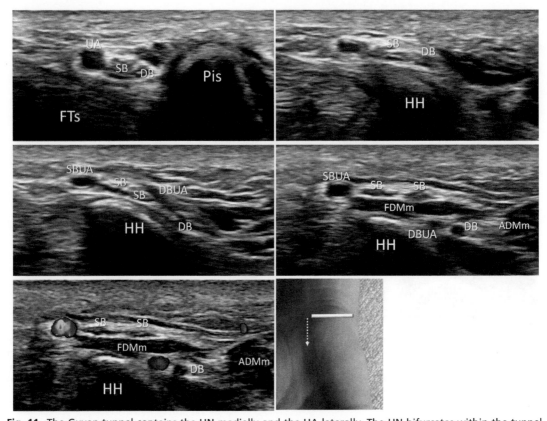

Fig. 11. The Guyon tunnel contains the UN medially and the UA laterally. The UN bifurcates within the tunnel, distal to the pisiform, in 2 terminal branches: SB and DB. The SB runs close to the UA, and the DB runs alongside to the hook of the hamate. Similarly, the UA splits into 2 branches—the SBUA and DBUA—following their respective nerves. ADMm, adductor digiti minimi muscle; DB, deep motor branch; DBUA, deep branch of ulnar artery; FDMm, flexor digiti minimi muscle; SB, sensory branch; SBUA, superficial branch of ulnar artery. Dotted arrow on artwork illustrates the axial progression of the probe from proximal to distal Guyon tunnel.

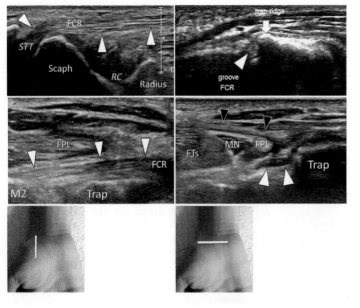

Fig. 12. The FCR (*white arrowheads*) courses in a separate fibrous tunnel made by an extension of the transverse carpal ligament (*black arrowheads*) inserted into the trapezial ridge (*arrow*). Then, the FCR reaches a groove situated on the ulnar side of the trapezium and inserts into the palmar aspect of the base of the second metacarpal. FCR, flexor carpi radialis; FPL, flexor pollicis longus; MN, median nerve; STT, scaphotrapezoid-trapezium joint; Trap, trapezium.

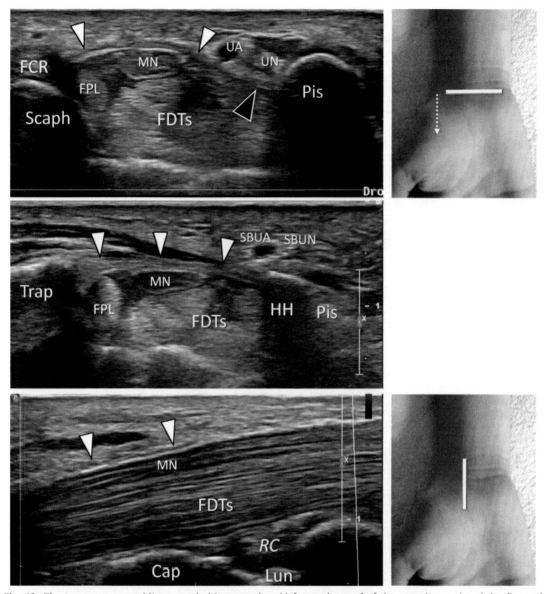

Fig. 13. The transverse carpal ligament (*white arrowheads*) forms the roof of the carpal tunnel and the floor of the Guyon tunnel (*black arrowhead*). Proximally, the carpal tunnel is delineated by the scaphoid at its radial side and the pisiform at its ulnar side. These bones appear as round hyperechoic structures with posterior acoustic shadows. Distally, the carpal tunnel is delineated by the trapezium at its radial side and the hook of the hamate at its ulnar side. The trapezium is characterized by its flat palmar surface, and the hook of the hamate is characterized by its short curvilinear shape. Because of the more central location of the hook of the hamate, the size of the distal tunnel is smaller than the proximal one. Within the carpal tunnel, the MN is located superficial to the FDTs and on the ulnar side of the FPL. FDTs, flexor digitorum tendons. Dotted arrow on artwork illustrates the axial progression of the probe from proximal to distal carpal.

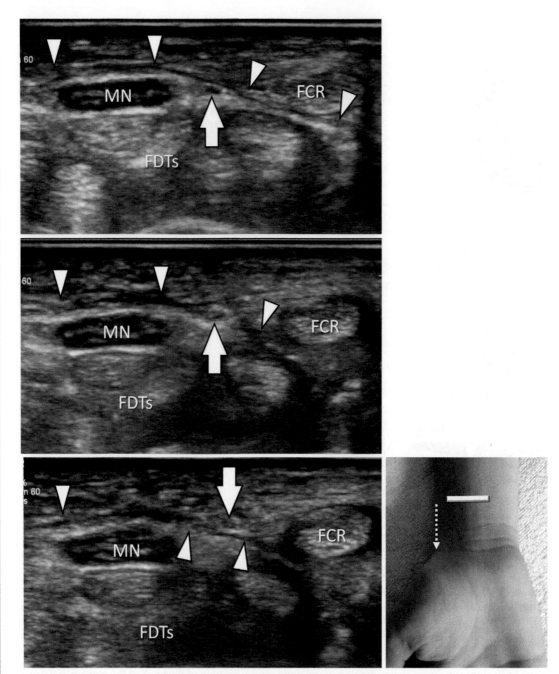

Fig. 14. The palmar cutaneous branch (*arrows*) of the MN arises from its palmar-radial quadrant, cranial to the proximal wrist crease. Then, it pierces the antebrachial fascia or the transverse carpal ligament (*arrowheads*), close to the FCR tendon. The dotted arrow indicates the progression of the probe from proximal to distal wrist.

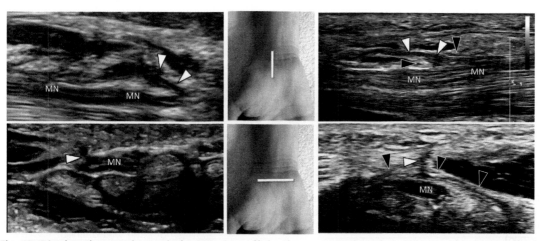

Fig. 15. Distal to the carpal tunnel, the MN gives off the thenar motor branch (*white arrowheads*). The classic extraligamentous course of the thenar branch is illustrated on the left US images. The transligamentous course of the thenar branch (*black arrowheads*), illustrated on the right US images, is seen in less than 4% of the population.

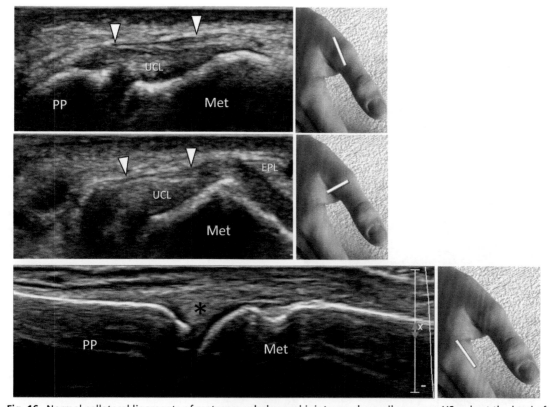

Fig. 16. Normal collateral ligaments of metacarpophalangeal joints may be easily seen on US only at the level of the thumb, the radial aspect of the second metacarpophalangeal joint, and the ulnar aspect of the fifth metacarpophalangeal joint. The ulnar collateral ligament (UCL) of the metacarpophalangeal joint of the thumb appears as a hyperechoic structure joining the first metacarpal to the proximal phalanx. Superficial to this ligament, the adductor pollicis muscle aponeurosis is visualized (*white arrowheads*). The radial collateral ligament of the second finger is illustrated as a thick hyperechoic structure (*asterisk*) close to the bone. Met, metacarpal; PP, proximal phalanx.

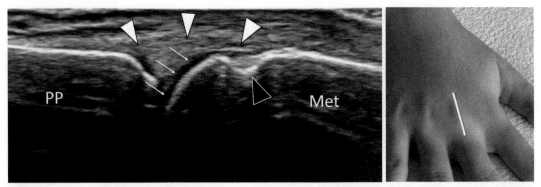

Fig. 17. In a longitudinal US view of the dorsal hand, the normal dorsal metacarpal notch (*black arrowhead*), measuring 0.7 to 2.2 mm, should not be confused with an erosion. The dorsal metacarpal synovial recess thickness (*white arrowheads*) should not exceed 2.2 mm. Fine hypoechoic cartilage covers the metacarpal head (*small arrows*).

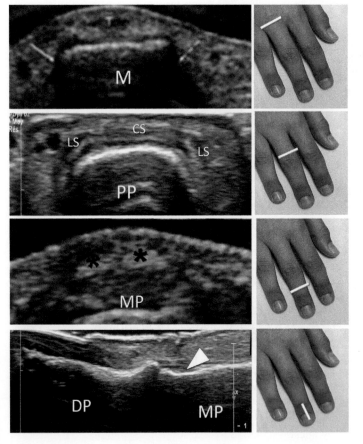

Fig. 18. Over the dorsal hand, the 4 tendons of the extensor digitorum muscle pass over the dorsal aspect of the metacarpal bones to reach the respective fingers. At the level of the metacarpal, the extensor tendon is covered by the sagittal band (*arrowhead*). At the level of the proximal phalanx, the extensor tendon divides into a central slip (CS) and 2 lateral slips (LSs). The CS inserts into the base of the middle phalanx, whereas the LSs (*asterisk*) fuse at the level of the MP to insert into the base of the distal phalanx. DP, distal phalanx; MP, middle phalanx.

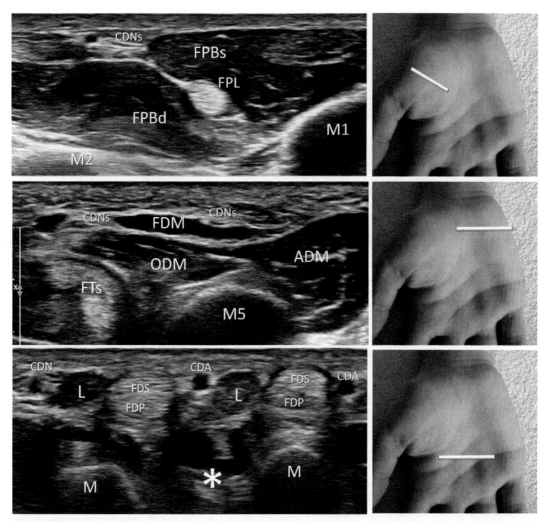

Fig. 19. At the thenar side of the palm, the most lateral flexor tendon is the FPL tendon. This tendon courses between the FPBs and FPBd heads of the FPBm. In the middle palm, the axial view displays the FDS and FDP. On each side of the tendons are located the common digital arteries and nerves and the lumbrical muscles. More deeply, the interosseous muscles (*asterisk*) are seen filling the space between the metacarpals. At the hypothenar side of the palm are situated the adductor digiti minimi (ADM), flexor digiti minimi (FDM), and opponent digiti minimi (ODM) muscles. CDA, common digital artery; CDN, common digital nerve; FDP, flexor digitorum profundus; FDS, flexor digitorum superficialis; FPBd, flexor pollicis brevis, deep head; FPBs, flexor pollicis brevis, superficial head; M1 to M5 first to fifth metacarpal.

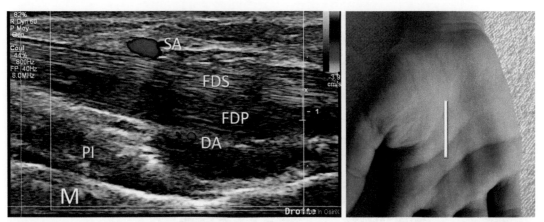

Fig. 20. In the palm, the SA lies superficial to the flexor tendons and is well demonstrated with color Doppler US; the DA is not always clearly identified at the level of the metacarpals and the palmar interosseous muscles. PI, palmar interosseous; SA, superficial arterial arch.

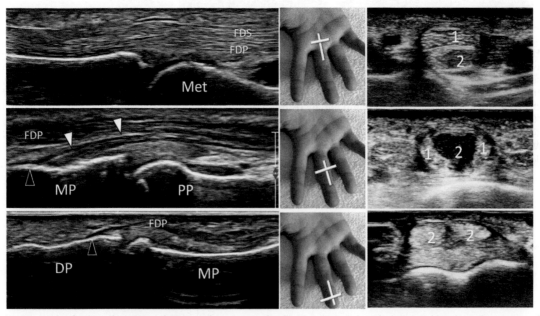

Fig. 21. In the fingers, the FDP and FDS tendons run in the fibrous digital sheath delimited by the volar aspect of the phalangeal cortex and the digital pulleys. When the FDS enters the digital sheath, it splits into 2 tendons (1) to surround the FDP (2). Then, the FDS inserts into the middle phalanx (*white arrowheads*) and the FDP continues toward the distal phalanx and inserts into its base (*black arrowhead*).

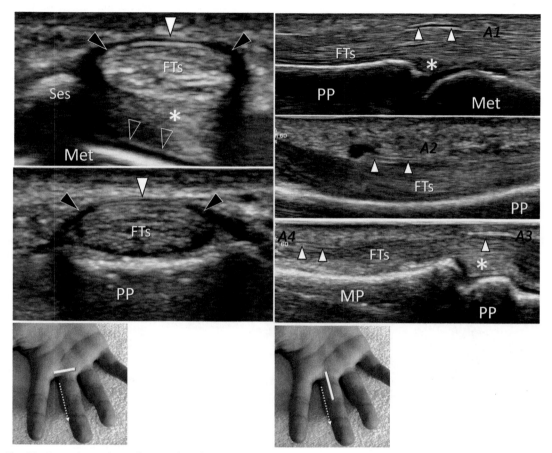

Fig. 22. Normal annular pulleys are less than 1 mm thick. The pulleys are usually hyperechoic when perpendicular to the US beam (*white arrowheads*) and hypoechoic laterally (*black arrowheads*). Dynamic scanning during flexion and extension of the finger illustrates the stationary pulley system from the underlying gliding tendons. Palmar plates (*asterisk*) lie between the FTs and the metacarpal and phalangeal heads. A palmar plate appears normally as a hyperechoic structure, with a rectangular shape on the axial view (see also **Fig. 23**). The articular cartilage (*white empty arrowheads*) is seen as a fine and regular hypoechoic curved line covering the hyperechoic subchondral bone. A sesamoid is observed as a bright rounded structure with a posterior acoustic shadow at the level of the metacarpophalangeal joint. A1 to A4, first to fourth annular pulley; FTs, flexor tendons; Ses, sesamoid.

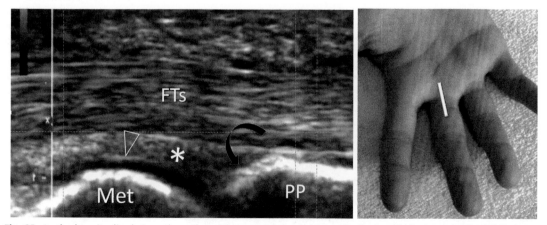

Fig. 23. In the longitudinal view, the palmar plate appears as a triangular hyperechoic structure (*asterisk*), inserting into the base of the phalanx (*curved arrow*) and pointing cranially. The articular cartilage (*white empty arrowhead*) is clearly visible.

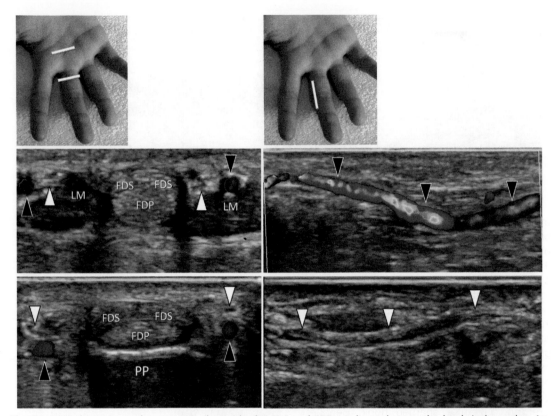

Fig. 24. Digital arteries and nerves run alongside the FDS and FDP tendons, close to the lumbrical muscles. Arteries, usually smaller than the adjacent veins, are better identified with color Doppler US (*black arrowheads*). Nerves (*white arrowheads*) are recognizable by their fascicular appearance. LM, lumbrical muscle.

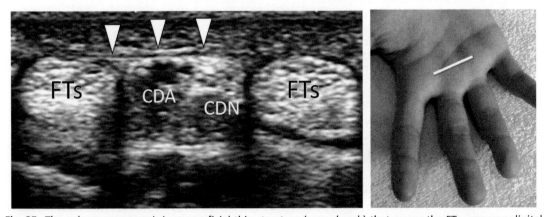

Fig. 25. The palmar aponeurosis is a superficial thin structure (*arrowheads*) that covers the FTs, common digital arteries, and common digital nerves of the palm.

similarly. Normal typical images are presented together with inserts indicating the position or the course of the transducer.

Wrist (**Figs. 1–16**).
Hand (**Figs. 17–25**).

CLINICS CARE POINTS

- Using high-quality equipment (high-frequency linear array transducers ranging from 10 to 15 MHz; adapted size and shape of the probe, like a hockey-stick probe; Doppler imaging; compound imaging; extended field-of-view imaging; steering-based imaging; 3-dimensional imaging; elastography; contrast media; and DICOM capacities for static and dynamic recording)

- Standardization of US examination technique, including first examination on the short axis and then on the long axis plane, dynamic evaluation, and correct focusing.

- Appropriateness of US indications, pertinent clinical information, and patient's history.

- Accurate interpretation of the images and correlation of the US findings with clinical data

- Use of x-rays when superficial cortical outgrowths or ingrowths are suspected

DISCLOSURES OF CONFLICTS OF INTEREST

V. Créteur disclosed no relevant relationships. A. Madani disclosed no relevant relationships. S. Bianchi disclosed no relevant relationships.

REFERENCES

1. Bianchi S, Martinoli C, Sureda D, et al. Ultrasound of the hand. Eur J Ultrasound 2001;14:29–34.

2. Créteur V, Peetrons P. Ultrasonography of the wrist and the hand. J Radiol 2000;81:346–52.

3. Lee JC, Healy JC. Normal sonographic anatomy of the wrist and hand. Radiographics 2005;25:1577–90.

4. Bianchi S, Martinoli C, Abdelwahab F. High-frequency ultrasound examination of the wrist and hand. Skeletal Radiol 1999;28:121–9.

5. Chiavaras MM, Jacobson JA, Yablon CM, et al. Pitfalls in wrist and hand ultrasound. AJR Am J Roentgenol 2014;203:531–40.

6. Catalano O, Roldán FA, Varelli C, et al. Skin cancer: findings and role of high-resolution ultrasound. J Ultrasound 2019;22:423–31.

7. Morvan G, Brasseur J-L, Sans N. Superficial US of superficial bones. J Radiol 2005;86:1892–903.

8. Créteur V, Borens B, Bouchaibi SE, et al. Osteolytic femoral lesion detected by sonography in a case of light chain deposition disease. J Clin Ultrasound 2014;42:444–8.

9. Bianchi S. Ultrasound and bone: a pictorial review. J Ultrasound 2020;23(3):227–57.

10. Peetrons P. Ultrasound of muscles. Eur Radiol 2002; 12:35–43.

11. Martinoli C, Bianchi S, Dahmane M, et al. Ultrasound of tendons and nerves. Eur Radiol 2002; 12:44–55.

12. Gitto S, Draghi F. Normal sonographic anatomy of the wrist with emphasis on assessment of tendons, nerves, and ligaments. J Ultrasound Med 2016;35: 1081–94.

13. Moraux A, Vandenbossche L, Demondion X, et al. Anatomical study of the pisotriquetral joint ligaments using ultrasonography. Skeletal Radiol 2012;41:321–8.

14. Créteur V, Bacq C, Widelec J. Sonography of peripheral nerves-first part: upper limb. J Radiol 2004;85:1887–99.

15. Petrover D, Bellity J, Vigan M, et al. Ultrasound imaging of the thenar motor branch of the median nerve: a cadaveric study. Eur Radiol 2017;27: 4883–8.

16. Bianchi S, J-Beaulieu Y, Poletti P-A. Ultrasound of the ulnar-palmar region of the wrist : normal anatomy and anatomic variations. J Ultrasound 2020;23(3): 349–62.

17. Créteur V, Madani A, Gosset N. Apport de l'échographie dans la maladie de Dupuytren. J Radiol 2010; 91:687–91.

18. Draghi F, Gitto S, Bianchi S. Injuries to the collateral ligaments of the metacarpophalangeal and interphalangeal joints. J Ultrasound Med 2018;37(9): 2117–33.

19. Bianchi S, Gitto S, Draghi F. Ultrasound features of trigger finger review of the literature. J Ultrasound Med 2019;38(12):3141–54.

20. Bianchi S, Becciolini M. Ultrasound evaluation of sesamoid fractures of the hand. J Ultrasound Med 2019;38:1913–20.

21. Créteur VM, Durieux PF, Cuylits N. Case 247: Jersey finger of the fifth finger. Radiology 2017;285:683–9.

Sonography, My Personal Assistant at Hand Outpatient Clinic

Samuel Christen, MD[a], Esther Vögelin, MD[b],*

KEYWORDS

- Clinical impact • Sonographic diagnosis • Hand • Wrist • Ultrasound

KEY POINTS

- Ultrasonography is an important diagnostic tool in the daily practice of a hand surgeon in evaluating traumatic and degenerative lesions of bones, joints, ligaments, tendons, annular pulleys, nerves, and vessels; detection of foreign bodies; and evaluation of small tumors.
- Ultrasonography offers an internal image of anatomic structures in axial, coronal, and transversal planes as well as observing dynamic changes during motion.
- Ultrasonography is examiner dependent but allows a direct, noninvasive view of anatomic structures in the best suitable way of the examiner with regard to the pathology of the patient.
- Ultrasonography immediately allows to infiltrate precisely in joint or tendon spaces, to plan surgery, or to perform sonographically assisted miniinvasive surgery.

 Video content accompanies this article at http://www.hand.theclinics.com.

INTRODUCTION

Ultrasonography (US) is an easily accessible, rapid, radiation-free, noninvasive imaging technique with useful dynamic capabilities suitable to study small (<3 cm) and superficial structures. If a lesion is previously suspected at clinical assessment US may add useful information confirming or modifying the diagnostic and therapeutic path. In the literature, US has been shown to confirm the diagnosis in 40% of patients with a history of previous trauma, 21% with a history of overuse, 16% after previous surgery, 13% with a history of neuropathy, and in 10% with diffuse pain.[1] However, most of the patients with hand problems are still referred to radiologists, rheumatologists, or neurologists who perform US and then send back the patient to the referring institution with a delay of possible treatment. Using US in the hands of the treating physician, a direct patient feedback and history during examination is available influencing a possible immediate treatment. In examination of tendon and ligamentous injuries, dynamic imaging can be obtained, which is invaluable in the assessment of annular pulley injuries, joint stability, and tendon subluxations or adhesions. With the use of a high-frequency linear array transducer in the range of 15 to 18 MHz, imaging of all interesting structures in both longitudinal and cross-sectional axes is available. It is important to learn to interpret lateral spatial resolution, tissue contrast, and posterior shadowing as well as to decrease artifacts related to reverberation and noise. In soft tissue masses, inflammatory or infectious tenosynovitis, color and power Doppler imaging may demonstrate hyperemic conditions differentiating granulation tissue, hypervascular tumors, or arteriovenous fistulae.[2] With the following case series, I would like to demonstrate the advantage of US in the hands of the treating physician for the patient in order to

[a] Hand, Plastic and Reconstructive Surgery, Cantonal Hospital St. Gallen, Rorschacherstrasse 95, 9007 St.Gallen, Switzerland; [b] Hand Surgery and Surgery of Peripheral Nerves, Plastic and Surgery, Inselspital, University Hospital of Bern, Freiburgstrasse 10, CH-3010 Bern, Switzerland
* Corresponding author.
E-mail address: esther.voegelin@insel.ch

Hand Clin 38 (2022) 19–29
https://doi.org/10.1016/j.hcl.2021.08.002

diagnosis the problem immediately, to initiate conservative treatment such as precise infiltration or to plan surgery without any delay.

Traumatic Disorders of Bones, Joints, and Tendons

Ultrasound has additive value in diagnosis of minimally displace fracture with high sensitivity and specificity.[3] We started to use it in suspicion of fractures such as subcapital metacarpal, scaphoid, or phalangeal fractures as a first or additional diagnostic tool. US may identify fractures shadowed by adjacent bones.[4] Osseous structures including avulsed fragments can be distinctively recognized by their pronounced posterior acoustic shadow and strongly reflective hyperechoic surface. Acute nondisplaced fractures appear as a focal hypoechoic interruption with an otherwise hyperechoic cortex. For a patient, it may be important to diagnose a nondisplaced fracture (**Fig. 1**, Video 1), especially when this fracture is not visible on anteroposterior or lateral conventional radiograph. US helped to initiate conservative functional treatment with buddy taping without the necessity to perform a computed tomography (CT) scan or a dynamic radiograph to check the stability of the present fracture pattern.

With US the extent of intraarticular osseous avulsion injuries of small joints (interphalangeal and metacarpal phalangeal joints) may be assessed. In proximal interphalangeal joint dislocation, US allows to localize preoperatively the intraarticular fragments in relation to the collateral ligaments as in this example (**Fig 2**, Video 2). It was possible to differentiate the cause of joint instability by the osseous dislocated fragment from the radial side of the middle phalanx and not by ligament disruption or avulsion and an additional fracture. With the preoperative US information, surgery is better planable, also in more complex injuries involving the palmar plate, pulleys as well as osseous avulsion of the central slip.[5]

A common injury involves the ulnar collateral ligament (UCL) at the level of the first metacarpophalangeal (MCP) joint. The torn UCL may retract proximally allowing the overlying tendinous aponeurosis of the adductor pollicis muscle to slip underneath its proximal margin, forming the so-called Stener lesion and hindering nonoperative healing. US may identify not only a Stener lesion but allows to differentiate nondisplaced from displaced UCL tears and to distinguish partial tears from complete tears.[6] A ligamentous sprain is seen as diffuse hypoechoic thickening without focal disruption, whereas tears are seen as a discrete hypoechoic partial or complete discontinuity within the thickened ligament. With a Stener lesion, the UCL is retracted and balled-up proximally due to displacement by the interposed adductor aponeurosis (**Fig 3**, Video 3). The smooth outline of the thin hyperechoic adductor aponeurosis will be identified distal and deep to the proximally retracted UCL in a transversal US scan. Partial or full-thickness ligament tears have immediate consequences for conservative or surgical treatment.

Similar to collateral ligament injury, partial tearing of the palmar plate manifests with

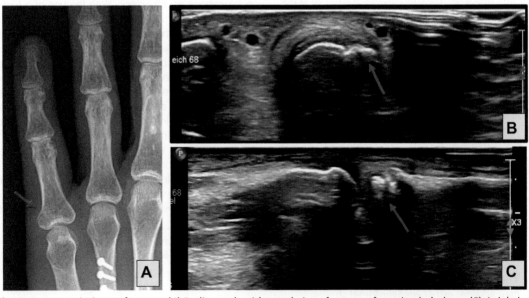

Fig. 1. Arrows pointing to fracture. (*A*) Radiograph without obvious fracture of proximal phalanx. (*B*) Axial view of dorsoulnar fracture. (*C*) Longitudinal view of dorsal fracture.

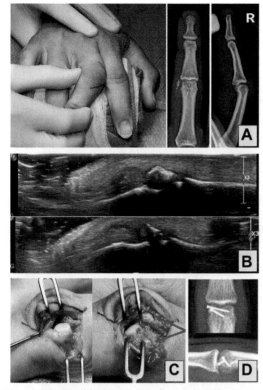

Fig. 2. (A) Unstable PIP joint, radiograph with osseous avulsion injury of radial collateral ligament. (B) Longitudinal view of US with intraligament fracture fragment from the base of middle phalanx. (C) Intraoperative 1 mm screw fixation of the thin fragment at the base of middle phalanx with partially divided collateral ligament (arrows). (D) Postoperative radiograph.

hypoechoic edematous thickening. Complete tears occur at the distal insertion and will appear as focal structural discontinuity with pericapsular edema and fluid.[7] Accompanying intraarticular avulsion fractures commonly occur, appearing as a hyperechoic focus with prominent posterior acoustic shadowing adjacent to the PIP joint. Partial and complete osseous avulsion of the palmar plate as well as its stability and stiffness including the subcutaneous edema in the involved digit may be assessed by US after trauma (Fig 4, Video 4). According to the US findings, the treatment plan may be adapted. With a sonographically and clinically stable palmar plate, a splint in extension may be used instead of an extension-stop-splint, to avoid flexion contracture. According to the edema seen in US early and in due course, local compression bandages (Coban) or lymph-tapes may be used to reduce swelling.[8]

US has proved utility in assessing the extent of tendon discontinuity and retraction as well as adhesion formation and in identifying associated osseous avulsion injuries or multitendon injury. In this case with complete inability to flex the finger after a proximal phalanx fracture, only US could demonstrate which flexor tendon (superficial, deep tendon) was involved and whether there was a rupture with a gap or rather posttraumatic adhesions (Fig 5, Video 5 + 6). The probability of a 1-stage or 2-stage tendon reconstruction compared with a tenolysis could be estimated, and the patient was accordingly informed.

With careful attention to scanning technique and anatomic detail, partial tendon tears can be

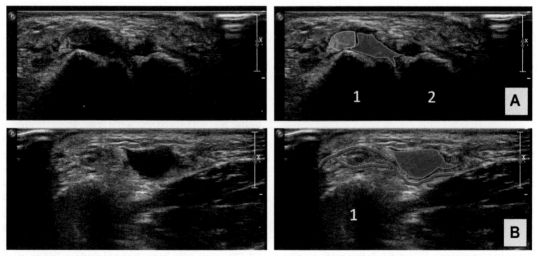

Fig. 3. (A) Longitudinal view of the head of MC I and basis of proximal phalanx I. Green = proximal UCL stump. Blue = hematoma, red line = adductor aponeurosis. (B) Transversal view of the head of MC I; red line = adductor aponeurosis with sagittal band and extensor tendon (Stener lesion); blue = hematoma over adductor aponeurosis. MC, metacarpal.

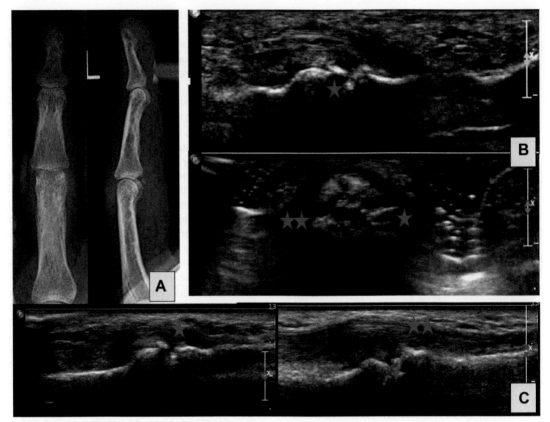

Fig. 4. (A) Palmar plate avulsion, little fragment on radiograph. (B) Radial palmar plate fragment* with 1 mm dehiscence from base of middle phalanx, longitudinal, and additional small impression on ulnar side** in axial view. (C) Radial* and ulnar** stable fragments after 5 months.

quantified, aiding in surgical planning. Postoperative repair sites may demonstrate lasting attritional changes and loss of the normal hyperechoic fibrillar pattern due to granulation tissue and scarring, complicating the assessment for reinjury.[9] Noting the presence or absence of secondary signs such as surrounding edema and fluid as well as using real-time dynamic techniques to directly evaluate morphologic integrity is useful in distinguishing chronic injury.

Degenerative Disorders of Joints and Tendons

Wrist

Although conventional radiography is the current referenced standard imaging modality for evaluation of bone changes (osteophytes subchondral sclerosis, cysts, and joint space narrowing), US has been proved more sensitive than conventional radiography in detecting certain bone changes and joint space narrowing.[10] Painful degenerative wrist conditions include lesions such as scapholunate advanced collapse conditions. In this 50-year-old lady with massive wrist pain after monotonic

laboratory work, radiograph and CT scan demonstrated an osteophyte at the dorsal horn of the lunate bone. Only US demonstrated the localization of the osteophyte dorsal to the SL ligament toward the midcarpal joint and indicated the surgical procedure including diagnostic arthroscopy and mini-arthrotomy to remove the osteophyte without the necessity of SL ligament reconstruction (**Fig 6**, Video 7).

In this other painful swollen wrist after overuse of the hand a week ago, it was necessary to discriminate an inflammatory wrist condition from an infection. Sonographically, fluid was detected in the radiocarpal joint apart from hyperechogenic changes also in the triangular fibrocartilage complex (TFCC) joint (**Fig 7**), assuming calcium pyrophosphate deposition (CPPD) deposits. With US even small deposits of CPPD, with high specificity and sensitivity, and no irradiation risks can be detected. This is important, especially because CPPD generally may be present in more than one joint and not strictly related to clinical presentation. The hyperechoic spots are the most frequent US pattern, and fibrocartilage is more

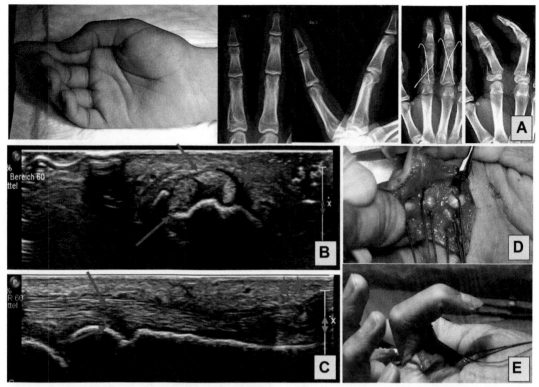

Fig. 5. (A) No active flexion of index finger 5 months after removal of K-wires for fixing proximal phalanx fractures II and III. (B) Radial FDS and FDP (*arrows*) adherent to fracture site in axial view. *Ulnar FDS tendon slip. (C) No discontinuation of tendons in longitudinal view but accordion phenomenon** due to tenodesis at fracture site. (D) Intraoperative adherence of radial FDS and FDP tendon at fracture site. (E) After tenolysis. FDP, flexor digitorum profundus; FDS, flexor digitorum superficialis.

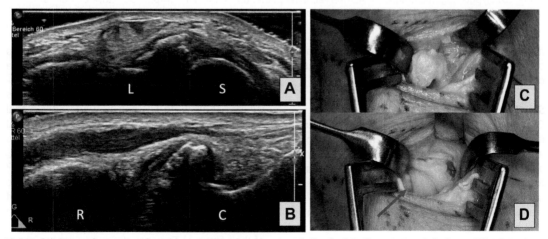

Fig. 6. (A) Osteophyte over dorsal horn of lunate dorsal and distal of SL ligament, axial plane. (B) Osteophyte over midcarpal joint at capitate, longitudinal plane. (C) Intraoperative view of osteophyte over dorsal horn of lunate. (D) Arrow at intact SL interval. SL, scapholunate.

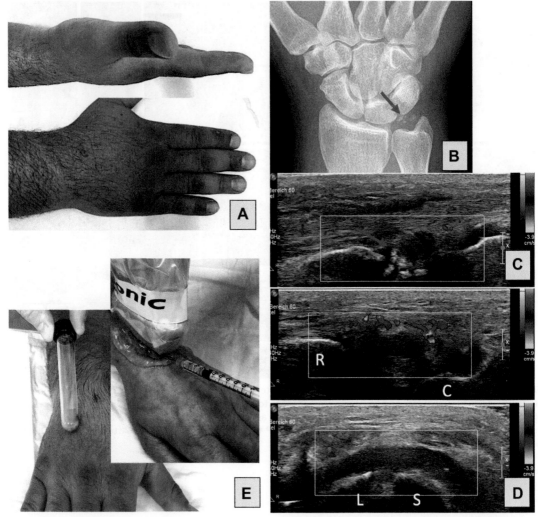

Fig. 7. (*A*) Swelling at wrist and dorsum of the hand without trauma. (*B*) Hyperechogenic changes (*arrow*) in radiograph. (*C*) Hyperechogenic spots (*arrow*) and hypervascularity radiocarpal and midcarpal, longitudinal plane. (*D*) Hypoechogenic fluid over SL interval, axial plane. (*E*) Sterile sonographic puncture of fluid at dorsal radiocarpal joint, crystals confirmed by microscopy, bacterial infection excluded.

frequently affected compared with the hyaline cartilage. The presence of CPPD crystals is usually confirmed by microscopy.[11]

Small joints

Disruption of the sagittal bands or juncturae tendinum results mainly in ulnar subluxation due to preferential tearing of the radial-sided sagittal band[12] after a closed trauma or spontaneously in rheumatoid arthritis. The dynamic, real-time capabilities of ultrasound are of great utility in establishing the diagnosis. Discontinuity, asymmetric thickening, and hypoechogenicity of the paramedian sagittal band may be seen particularly well on short-axis views through the MCP region (**Fig 8**, Video 8 + 9) in this young lady with rheumatoid arthritis.

US revealed a lesion of the radial sagittal bands and attenuation but not a rupture of the juncturae tendinum.[13] Because of the attenuation and general laxity of the tissue, surgical treatment was initiated. Follow-up US can be used after a trial of nonoperative immobilization therapy or surgical repair to evaluate the integrity of the sagittal bands and assess for residual radial/ulnar instability.

Lesions to the collateral ligaments of the MCP joints are less common in the fingers than in the thumb. The slightly hypoechoic appearance of the normal collateral ligaments may be due to an artifact and may be related to the oblique course of their fibers.[14] They are difficult to assess especially in central rays. In this patient (**Fig 9**, Video 10), US was helpful to diagnose the prominent

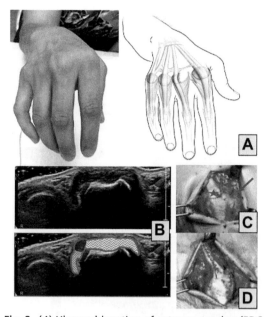

changes in the involved radial collateral ligament in comparison to the ligaments of the neighbor finger. Chronic steroid infiltration resulted in an instability of the radial collateral ligament of the middle finger but not in the index finger. Hyperechogenic changes with US proposed a chondrocalcinosis and a thickened ligament appearance but no interruption. The clinical snapping and the instability of the central digit suggested an incompetent ligament. However, with US only the dorsal and palmar aspects of the ligament of central rays may be assessed but not the hole ligament course, demonstrating one of the limitations of US.

Tendons

Similarly, suppurative tenosynovitis manifest often with internal fluid, capsular/sheath thickening, and hyperemia. Although the appearance is closely mimicked by noninfectious, inflammatory tendinopathy, the clinical context, presentation, and laboratory findings are frequently discriminatory. Fluid sampling and drainage is typically warranted when the cause remains indeterminate to exclude purulent infection,[15] as seen in the following patient with a chronic swelling 5 weeks after A1 pulley release in the middle finger (**Fig 10**). Sonographic findings of rheumatoid tenosynovitis include thickening of the tendon sheath, intrasynovial fluid, and alterations in the tendon echo texture

Fig. 8. (A) Ulnar subluxation of extensor tendon (EDC III, *arrow*) of middle finger. (B) Axial plane of extensor tendon hood with ulnar subluxation and scarring of both attenuated and ruptured sheath of sagittal bands. (C) Attenuated external sheath (*arrow*), subluxated EDC III*. (D) Repaired, recentered extensor hood by strip of proximal EDC III. EDC, *extensor* digitorum communis.

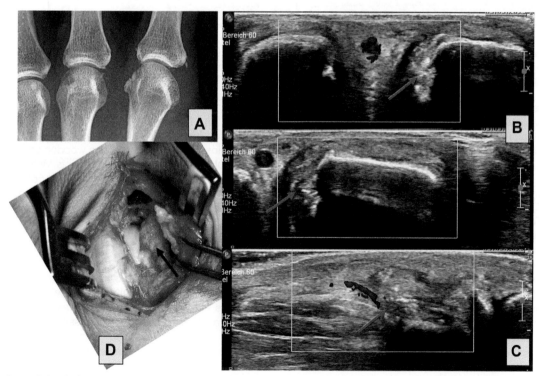

Fig. 9. (A) Calcifications in the radial collateral ligament (CL) origin at MCP III, ulnar and radial CL at MCP II. (B) Calcification and thickening of radial CL at MCP III (*arrow*), axial plane. (C) Longitudinal plane of thickened CL at radial MCP III (*arrow*). (D) Complete destruction (*arrow*) of radial collateral CL at MCP III, intact EDC III, cartilage, and sagittal bands.

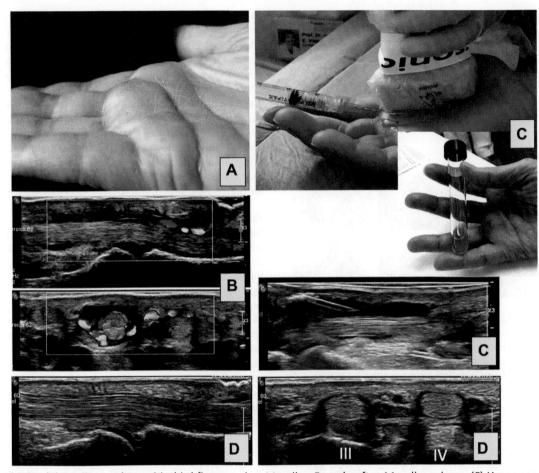

Fig. 10. (A) Swelling and synovitis third finger and at A1 pulley, 5 weeks after A1 pulley release. (B) Hypervascularity and an echogenic fluid around flexor tendons of third finger, longitudinal and axial plane. (C) Sterile puncture of synovial fluid sonographically controlled, bacterial infection excluded. (D) Five months later normal appearance of A1 pulley and tendons longitudinal and axial.

ranging from diffuse blurring to focal defects. Doppler imaging reveals synovial hyperemia as a sign of active inflammation; a decrease in synovial vascularization indicates fibrous pannus formation as well as a good response to treatment.[16]

Lumps and Bumps

Foreign bodies

US, with its high sensitivity, is an excellent first-line imaging modality to analyze tumors and foreign bodies. Depending on surface characteristics and composition, foreign bodies will have a generally hyperechoic imaging appearance with variable acoustic shadowing. In the case of glass or metal fragments, reverberation artifact and dirty acoustic shadowing are found. Abscess or granuloma formation may occur in subacute to chronic cases, appearing respectively as an ill-defined hypoechoic halo surrounding the central foreign body locus or as a complex heterogeneous fluid collection

with peripheral mural hypervascularity.[17] In this patient (**Fig 11**, Video 11), chronic swelling and decreased motion of his index finger over 2 years after a closed trauma caused by a wooden splinter encapsulated by granulation tissue is detected with US. The rather weird localization of the splinter including the granulation tissue dorsoradially to the flexor tendons and the A2 pulley demonstrated by US helped to plan surgery accordingly.

Soft tissue mass

Posttraumatic vascular anomalies presenting as tumors in the adult population are rare and may occur as extravascular and or intravascular pyogenic granulomas. With US, it is possible to differentiate highly vascularized tumors such as granulation tissue from tumors with changes in the vascular flow of an intravascular pyogenic granuloma or a venous malformation. US demonstrates a hypoechoic mass with monophasic

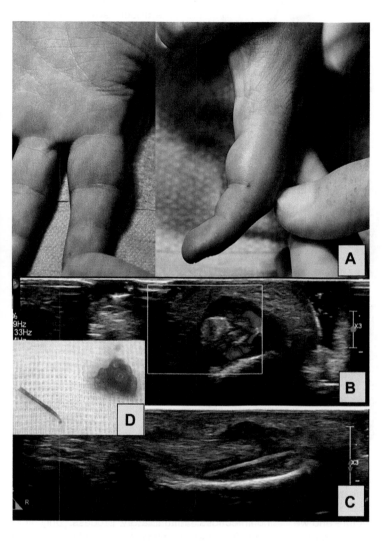

Fig. 11. (*A*) Chronic swelling proximal phalanx of left index finger 2 years after closed trauma. (*B*) Granulation tissue dorsoradial of flexor tendons, axial plane of proximal phalanx. (*C*) Longitudinal plane with foreign body dorsoulnar of flexor tendons. (*D*) Surgery revealed wooden splinter (10 × 1 mm), granulation tissue.

low-velocity flow or occasionally no flow with the Doppler mode.[18] If there is flow within these tumors, a vascular venous or arterial signal using color Doppler may indicate an arteriovenous fistula feeding the tumor as in this patient (**Fig 12**). Vascular malformations present sonographically as hypervascular tumors with an arterial or venous flow differentiating from hypervascular tumor without flow such as granuloma tissue. The subcutaneous mass around the PIP joint in this patient was diagnosed by US as a vascular malformation tumor due to the Doppler signal and surgery with looking for a vascular stalk feeding the tumor could be planned.

DISCUSSION

US has the potential to affect diagnostic thinking and therapeutic management, especially in a posttraumatic setting but also in degenerative lesions. Sonography plays a pivotal role in the management of inflammatory, traumatic, and neoplastic lesions of the hand and wrist. Good anatomic delineation, pathologic correlation, and the opportunity to perform procedures using real-time imaging makes US the desirable imaging modality in the diagnosis and management of these lesions. The US technology therefore became an essential diagnostic tool in our daily practice for diagnosing posttraumatic sequelae, degenerative or overuse problems, planning surgeries, or even to perform precise infiltrations or sonographically assisted surgeries. US is appropriate for diagnosing superficial lesions, as they occur in the fingers and hand. It can discriminate cystic from solid lesions and identify tenosynovitis, vascular lesions, and foreign bodies. However, it requires a trained operator, and tissue characterization of other masses is often limited. If lesions overcome a size of more than 3 cm,

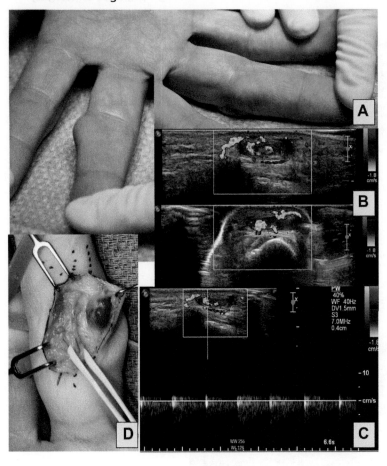

Fig. 12. (*A*) Progressive swelling with minimal tenderness on the radial side at the base of the middle phalanx after a small wound 6 months ago. (*B*) US color Doppler mode longitudinal and axial plane with vascularized tumor. (*C*) US color power Doppler arterial signal suggesting an arteriovenous connection within the tumor. (*D*) Intraoperative: vascular tumor, histologic pyogenic granuloma with a vascular stalk from the digital artery (*yellow band*).

they are more difficult to diagnose including the dignity but also the involvement of the surrounding tissue. Another limitation of US is the fact that we see only a certain depth of a structure and we do not get a complete 3-dimensional image from an anatomic structure as a bone or a joint or the TFCC, and this makes it difficult to assess collateral ligaments or the interosseous muscles of the hand in the central rays of the fingers from the dorsal to the palmar insertion. On the other hand, posttraumatic lesions are well demonstrated with US. We can look for fractures but it is only possible to judge one plane of a fracture at once (ie, lateral, posterior or anterior) in comparison to CT scans and MRI. Tendon injuries such as avulsion injuries of the flexus digitorum profundus (FDP), extensor tendon injuries, such as central slip or mallet fingers, sagittal band injuries, subluxation of tendons, pulley injuries, and ligamentous and volar plate injuries may be assessed dynamically by US. Foreign bodies may not only be localized but characterized whether there is a metal, glass, or wooden splinter. Inflammatory process or infections may be investigated by US. The presence of hyperemia on color or power Doppler imaging may

not always distinguish cellulitis from abscess, suppurative tenosynovitis, and or septic arthritis. Although the appearance is closely mimicked by noninfectious, inflammatory process, only fluid sampling and drainage is typically warranted when the cause remains indeterminate to exclude purulent infection.

SUMMARY

With the help of US in the outpatient clinics, traumatic and degenerative lesions are not only localized but the problem diagnosed and immediate conservative or surgical treatment initiated.

CLINICS CARE POINTS

- US is the third eye of hand surgery.
- Examiner-dependent examination in 3 planes, noninvasive.
- With US, precise infiltration of joints or tendon spaces and exact planning of surgical procedures.

DISCLOSURE STATEMENT

I hereby declare that I have no potential conflicts of interest to disclose.

SUPPLEMENTARY DATA

Supplementary data to this article can be found online at https://doi.org/10.1016/j.hcl.2021.08.002.

REFERENCES

1. Tagliafico A, Bignotti B, Rossi F, et al. Clinical Contribution of Wrist and Hand Sonography. J Ultrasound Med 2019;38:141–8.

2. Olubaniyi B, Bhatnagar G, Vardhanabhuti V, et al. Comprehensive musculoskeletal sonographic evaluation of the hand and wrist. J Ultrasound Med 2013;32:901–14.

3. Vreju F, Ciurea M, Popa D, et al. Ultrasonography in the diagnosis and management of noninflammatory conditions of the hand and wrist. Med Ultrasound 2016;18(1):90–5.

4. Hennecke B, Umbricht R, Vögelin E. „Top ten"-Indikationen zur Ultraschalldiagnostik an der Hand. Ther Umsch 2014;71(7):415–21.

5. Vögelin E. Ultrasonography: the third eye of hand surgeons. J Hand Surg 2020;45(3):219–25.

6. Melville D, Jacobson JA, Haase S, et al. Ultrasound of displaced ulnar collateral ligament tears of the thumb: the Stener lesion revisited. Skeletal Radiol 2013;42(5):667–73.

7. Rettig A. Athletic injuries of the wrist and hand: part II—overuse injuries of the wrist and traumatic injuries to the hand. Amj Sports Med 2004;32(1):262–73.

8. Leclère FM, Mathys L, Juon B, et al. The role of dynamic ultrasound in the immediate conservative treatment of volar plate injuries of the PIP Joint: A Series of 78 Patients. Plast Surg 2017;25(3):151–6.

9. Chun K, Cho K. Postoperative ultrasonograhy of the musculoskeletal system. Ultrasonography 2015;34:195–205.

10. Vele P, Simon S-P, Damian L, et al. Clinical and ultrasound findings in patients with calcium pyrophosphate dihydrate deposition disease. Med Ultrason 2018;20(2):159–63.

11. McMurtry J, Isaacs J. Extensor tendons injuries. Clin Sports Med 2015;34(1):167–80.

12. Chinchalkar SJ, Barker CA, Owsley B. Relationship between Juncturae tendinum and sagittal bands. J Hand Microsurg 2015;7(1):96–101.

13. Draghi F, Gitto S, Bianchi S. Injuries to the Collateral Ligaments of the Metacarpo-phalangeal and Interphalangeal Joints. J Ultrasound Med 2018;37:2117–33.

14. Padrez K, Bress J, Johnson B, et al. Bedside ultrasound identification of infectious flexor tenosynovitis in the emergency department. West J Emerg Med 2015;16(2):260–2.

15. Gitto S, Draghi AG, Draghi F. Sonography of Nonneoplastic Disorders of the Hand and Wrist tendons. J Ultrasound Med 2018;37:51–68.

16. Bianchi S, Della Santa D, Glauser T, et al. Sonography of masses of the wrist and hand. AJR Am J Roentgenol 2008;191:1767–75.

17. Stacy GS, Bonham J, Chang A, et al. Soft-Tissue Tumors of the Hand – Imaging Features. Can Assoc Radiol J 2020;71(2):161–73.

DISCLOSURE STATEMENT

I hereby declare that I have no potential conflicts of interest to disclose.

SUPPLEMENTARY DATA

Supplementary data to this article can be found online at https://doi.org/10.1016/j.cul.2021.06.002.

REFERENCES

Flexor Tendons Sonography

Thomas Apard, MD, FEBHS

KEYWORDS

• Ultrasound • Hand • Surgery • Finger • Tendon • Flexor • Tenosynovitis

KEY POINTS

- Ultrasonography is the best examination for flexor tendons disease or in postoperative conditions.
- Hand surgeons must be taught about the ultrasound to improve their skills for flexor tendons management.
- Dynamic and comparative examination is mandatory for flexor tendons.

 Video content accompanies this article at http://www.hand.theclinics.com.

INTRODUCTION

Ultrasonography is the best examination to explore the flexor tendons anatomy and disorders from the wrist to the digit. It is the only dynamic and comparative tool easily accessible for the surgeon.[1]

Indeed, ultrasonography is actually available in all the departments of your hospital: in the operating room with the anesthesiologists; in the hospitalization area, thanks to the radiologists; and in the emergency room with the traumatologist.

Recent innovations permit to see superficially (high-frequency probes), precisely (smaller probes), and with greater softwares for an effective Doppler mode.[2] The screens are smaller and more convenient as in the past In order to propose a better panel of machines for the practitioner from the pocket scan to the big machine with rollers.

All these evolutions involve a good exploration of the flexor tendons dynamically: passively, dynamically, and against resistance. This examination permits a good explanation of the pathology or the treatment to the patients. It is also very easy to conserve a picture or a video in a medicolegal file or to share with the colleagues.

HOW TO PERFORM ULTRASOUND SCANNING OF FLEXOR TENDONS?

Hand is placed in complete supination on the table, fingers tightened to conserve the gel on them. A lot of gel is mandatory to fill the small cavities of the palmar side of the joints.

A very high-frequency probe must be preferred (minimal 15 MHz) to see perfectly all the details just under the skin. The hockey-stick probes are interesting but not so convenient: a classic linear probe is able to show the other fingers in comparaison. In real life, it is not a necessity to buy another probe just for the fingers.

The ultrasound (US) examination must always be comparative and dynamic: the examiner must be able to flex the fingers passively in all the position of the probe. If it is not possible, you can place the finger and the probe into a bath and get an image without touching the skin.[3]

In a longitudinal view (« in plane scan »):

The flexor tendons are easy to see. Note immediately how the tendons are running like a Chinese dragon and not horizontally (as we think when we operate them). Another remark is that the flexor tendon of the thumb and the flexor tendons of

Ultrasound Hand Surgery Center, 2 rue de Tocqueville Versailles, France
E-mail address: thomasapard@echo-chirurgie-versailles.fr

Hand Clin 38 (2022) 31–34
https://doi.org/10.1016/j.hcl.2021.08.009
0749-0712/22/© 2021 Elsevier Inc. All rights reserved.

the fifth finger are not in the same axis than the finger. It is very important to look for the tendon among the screen and not looking at the hand.

The heads of the metacarpal and phalangeal bones are covered by the cartilage dome that is anechoic (black). The palmar ligament is isoechoic and always larger than a surgeon think (Video 1).

For the thumb examination, a good tip is to ask the patient to put his/her hand in prone position to lay down the thumb on the table.

In a transversal view (« out plane scan »):

The pulleys are not visible physiologically. The shadow artifact is an anisotropic vertical band at each side of the pulley (similar to quilts). The chiasma of flexor digitorum superficialis (FDS) tendons is very well explored at the first phalanx: the tendon is progressively divided into 2 parts and seem to envelop the flexor digitorum profundus (FDP) tendon to cover its deep side (Video 2).

Passively the 2 tendons are gliding without effort in the tendon sheath. An anomaly must be suspected if the tendons are not moving harmoniously when the examiner flex the distal phalanx.

Actively, the patient has to move slowly to analyze the movement. If the tendons have been repaired, it is simple to follow the sutures and their trajectory under the pulleys.

FLEXOR TENDON DISORDERS UNDER ULTRASOUND
Trigger Finger

Tenosynovitis of the flexor digitorum tendons may be the result of systemic disorders, such as rheumatoid arthritis and related conditions, mechanical stress, or infectious processes. The hallmarks of acute tenosynovitis of the flexor digitorum tendons are an increased amount of sheath fluid, which is seen as an anechoic collection surrounding the tendons without modification when pressing on the probe (Video 3). In subacute and chronic tenosynovitis, thickening of the synovial sheath may also be seen. The pain under the probe at the metacarpal head suspects a trigger finger. In flexion/extension of the finger, the A1 pulley is too small for the flexor tendons, and the FDS tendon seems to have difficulties to glide, which is not the case of the FDP tendon. Sometimes, a cyst is present at the distal part of the A1 pulley but then does not move with the FDS.

The association of Dupuytren contracture and trigger finger is common; the fibromatosis is isoechoic and not seen correctly ultrasonographically.

The Ganglia of the Pulley

Digital ganglia are fibrous-walled cystic lesions filled with mucoid fluid that develop on tendons or peritendinous structures. They are generally found at the volar aspect of the base of the finger, close to the annular pulleys (A1 or less frequently A2). They are caused by microtrauma to the digital annular pulley, which is followed by mucoid degeneration. The third and fourth fingers are the most commonly involved. US depicts these cysts as small anechoic lesions with no discernible wall and posterior acoustic shadowing. They extend along the lateral and medial aspects of the flexor tendons. Dynamic examination demonstrates smooth gliding movement of the flexor tendons that does not affect the size or position of digital ganglia. Occasionally, the A2-pulley can be visualized as a thin hyperechoic band lying between the tendons and the ganglion. The size of digital ganglia can vary over time due to alternating increases and decreases in the mucoid content. In general, size changes correlate well with the patient's symptoms. Color Doppler shows an absence of internal flow signals. It can be used to determine the relationship of the cystic lesion with the adjacent vessels.

Rupture of the A2 Pulley

Acute tears of the annular pulleys are among the most frequent lesions in elite climbers.[4] They most commonly involve the ring and middle fingers. Tears are commonly seen in free climbers who use hand grips in which the entire weight of the body is borne by a single finger. Excessive traction on the flexor tendons when the fingers are flexed tears the pulleys and causes anterior bowstringing of the tendons, which no longer lie against the bone plane. The A2-pulley ruptures more frequently than the A4-pulley, and A2 tears may be associated with rupture of the A3-pulley. If they are not diagnosed, complete pulley tears can lead to flexion contractures of the proximal interphalangeal joint with secondary osteoarthritis. In patients presenting with an acute tear, local swelling and pain frequently limit the physical examination. The differential diagnosis, which includes other posttraumatic conditions, such as tenosynovitis or a sprain of proximal interphalangeal joint, can be difficult in these cases, and imaging findings play a primary role. However, if the torn pulleys are difficult to detect by imaging, the diagnosis of complete pulley rupture can be made indirectly by demonstrating palmar bowstringing of the flexor tendons. US is the best tool to diagnose these lesions because a dynamic and comparative US scanning during active forced flexion can enhance visualization of the subluxation of tendons to the top. During dynamic longitudinal US scanning, the patient is asked to keep the finger slightly flexed with the metacarpophalangeal joint extended, whereas the examiner tries to extend it by gently pushing the fingertip. Transverse sonograms confirm volar bowstringing of the flexor tendons but usually add no significant information.

The site of maximal bowstringing helps identify which pulley is ruptured. In A2 pulley rupture, maximal volar displacement occurs over the proximal phalanx, whereas in A4 pulley tears, the bowstringing is chiefly observed over the middle phalanx. A hypoechoic rim surrounding the tendons (due to the accumulation of sheath fluid) can be seen in the acute phase as an expression of secondary traumatic tenosynovitis. Dynamic sonograms obtained during flexion/extension movements of the finger show smooth gliding of the flexor tendons and are useful in the assessment of the tendons. Color Doppler shows a slight peripheral flow signal in case of acute tear. In most of cases, a swelling is present under the probe where the rupture is complete, and the patient helps the examiner to localize the trauma.

Fig. 1 is an original water bath device to test the pulleys under ultrasound.

The Distal Avulsion of the Flexor Digitorum Profundus Tendon or Jersey Finger

The clinical examination shows obviously the incapacity of the distal phalanx to flex actively. Radiographs are mandatory to see a bone fracture of distal phalanx.

US is interesting for 3 reasons: (1) to explain to the patient what is going on (pain is not so bad and the patient needs to understand the gravity of the issue); (2) to confirm the diagnosis (differential diagnosis are algodystrophy, a pathology of the tendon gliding, and pain of the DIP joint.);

and (3) to localize the tendon's retraction to evaluate the prognosis related to vinculas (Video 4).

Even for an injury with a suspicion of flexor tendon injury, ultrasonography can be a useful tool to diagnose a complete or a partial one.[5]

Postoperative Ultrasound Scanning of the Sutured Flexor Tendon

Several diagnoses can be made in case of pain and edema after a sutured flexor tendon: septic tenosynovitis, algodystrophy, rupture of the suture, inflammatory scare, neuropathic pain of the digital nerve. Mode-B US or color Doppler can answer to all this questions. Nevertheless, the patient is at ease to see if the evolution is correct.

Giant-Cell Tumor of the Tendon Sheath

Giant-cell tumors of the tendon sheath are considered a localized form of pigmented villonodular synovitis. They represent the second most common space-occupying lesion of the hand that involves peritendinous tissues. It appears as a painless, slow-growing, solid extraarticular mass on the volar aspect of the fingers; lateral and circumferential extension is usually present. Typically, the giant-cell tumor lies adjacent to normal-appearing flexor tendons. On US, the tumor is seen as a hypoechoic mass with sharp margins. Unlike digital ganglia, giant-cell tumors of the tendon sheath have internal echoes and no posterior acoustic enhancement. Some exhibit internal vasculature at color and power Doppler imaging. US may reveal displacement of the digital arteries and cortical erosions of the phalanges secondary to pressure from the overlying lesion. After surgery, US can be useful in screening for local recurrences.

CLINICS CARE POINTS

- US is now available easily without side effect for all practitioners to explore flexor tendons. Hand surgeons must know how to settle the machine and perform it.
- US explores dynamically the flexor tendons and then, is the only examination that can precisely see tendons pathologies, tumor, and pulley ruptures.

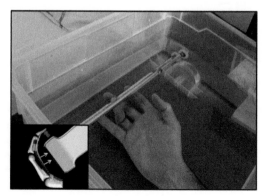

Fig. 1. In plane scanning of flexor tendons with A2 pulley. rupture: Red arrow illustrate the pression on the fingertip, yellow arrows illustrate the tendinous bowstringing.

DISCLOSURE

The authors have nothing to disclose.

SUPPLEMENTARY DATA

Supplementary data related to this article can be found online at https://doi.org/10.1016/j.hcl.2021.08.009.

REFERENCES

1. Apard T. Ultrasonography for the orthopaedic surgeon. Orthop Traumatol Surg Res 2019;105(1S):S7–14.
2. Soubeyrand M, Begin M, Pierrart J, et al. Ultrasonography for hand surgeons (lecture from the 46th meeting of French Society of Hand Surgery). Chir Main 2011;30(6):368–84.
3. Blaivas M, Lyon M, Brannam L, et al. Water bath evaluation technique for emergency ultrasound of painful superficial structures. Am J Emerg Med 2004;22(7):589–93.
4. Klauser A, Frauscher F, Bodner G, et al. Finger pulley injuries in extreme rock climbers: depiction with dynamic US. Radiology 2002;222(3):755–61.
5. Ravnic DJ, Galiano RD, Bodavula V, et al. Diagnosis and localisation of flexor tendon injuries by surgeon-performed ultrasound: a cadaveric study. J Plast Reconstr Aesthet Surg 2011;64:234–9.

Sonographic Diagnosis of Carpal Tunnel Syndrome

Sebastian Kluge, MD[a,b,*], Martin Langer, MD[c], Thomas Schelle, MD[d]

KEYWORDS

- Carpal tunnel syndrome • Sonography • Diagnostic ultrasound • Median nerve • Hand surgery

KEY POINTS

- Ultrasonographic diagnosis of carpal tunnel syndrome is mainly based on the assessment of the nerve cross-sectional area.
- Diagnostic ultrasound provides the ability to rule out secondary causes of nerve compression. However, a reliable assessment of the disease severity is not possible.
- Electrodiagnostic testing is based on the nerve's functional parameters. It therefore also allows estimation of the severity of the disease. It cannot be used to differentiate between causes of compression.
- Both diagnostic methods complement each other. In case of limitation to only one diagnostic method, the disadvantages of the specific technique become particularly noticeable postoperatively, especially when patients complain of persistent symptoms.
- Postoperative sonography does not provide functional parameters and therefore no clear comparison to preoperative measurements, while NCS does not provide information on the cause of persistent complaints.

 Video content accompanies this article at http://www.hand.theclinics.com.

INTRODUCTION

Carpal tunnel syndrome (CTS) is the most common compression neuropathy in humans and occurs idiopathically in 50% of cases. Patients aged between 40 and 60 years and women are significantly more often affected, in about 50% of cases, the disease occurs bilaterally.[1–5] The causes of the disease remain unclear. There is probably a multifactorial etiology. Possible causes include anatomic changes,[6–9] general disorders, increased strain, and also repetitive activities.[10,11] Secondary compression of the median nerve by flexor tendon synovitis also appears to have pathologic value.[12–15]

The diagnosis of CTS is based on typical clinical symptoms. Additional examinations are only used to confirm the clinical suspicion and complement each other.[16] Clinical symptoms usually consist of nocturnal or early morning tingling paresthesias in the distal supply area of the median nerve, from which the palmar cutaneous branch is typically excluded. Load-related and movement-related complaints are also possible and are usually associated with a flexed (Phalen's test) or extended position (reverse Phalen's test) of the wrist, in which the cross-sectional area of the carpal canal is additionally reduced. Advanced stages show a reduction of peripheral sensitivity and atrophy of the thenar prominence (**Fig. 1**).

[a] Handchirurgie Seefeld, Seefeldstrasse 27, Zurich 8008, Switzerland; [b] Department of Hand Surgery, Klinik Impuls, Bahnhofstraße 137, Wetzikon 8620, Switzerland; [c] Department of Trauma, Hand and Reconstructive Surgery, University of Munster, Waldeyerstraße 1, Munster 48149, Germany; [d] Department of Neurology, Klinikum Dessau-Rosslau, Auenweg 38, Dessau-Rosslau 06847, Germany
* Corresponding author. Handchirurgie Seefeld, Seefeldstrasse 27, Zurich 8008, Switzerland.
E-mail address: kluge@handchirurgie-seefeld.ch

Hand Clin 38 (2022) 35–53
https://doi.org/10.1016/j.hcl.2021.08.003

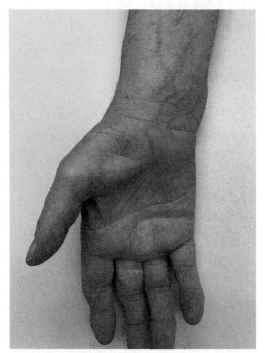

Fig. 1. Advanced carpal tunnel syndrome with atrophy of the thenar muscles.

In addition to confirming the clinical diagnosis, the additional apparative diagnostics also allow the assessment of the severity of the disease and the reliable differentiation from other, usually proximally localized compressions of the median nerve, which can clinically mimic CTS. However, legal aspects also play an important role, even if they usually only come into play in the event of postoperative complications or a lack of regeneration after decompression of the nerve.

Electrodiagnostic testing still represents the gold standard in confirmatory diagnostics. It provides information about the severity of the lesion (demyelinating vs axonal) and, when used correctly, can exclude other diseases that mimic CTS (eg, polyneuropathy). In cases of persistent postoperative symptoms, it helps decisively in objectifying a worsening of findings. The determination of the distal motor latency of the median nerve (in comparison to the ulnar nerve) as well as the comparative determination of the sensory nerve conduction velocity of the median nerve to the middle finger and the ulnar nerve to the small finger are routinely performed. The sensitivity and specificity of this method are 89% and 98%, respectively.[17] Specific conduction techniques can increase the sensitivity and specificity to 97.5% each.[18]

ESSENTIALS OF SONOGRAPHIC DIAGNOSTICS

Nerve compression results in a characteristic cascade of pathophysiologic changes consisting of endoneural edema, demyelination, axon degeneration, inflammation, fibrosis, resprouting of axons, and remyelination.[19] Many of these processes occur at the microcellular level and can only be objectified indirectly. However, some of these changes can be visualized quantitatively and semiquantitatively using appropriate imaging techniques.

Semiquantitative Criteria of Nerve Compression

Microvascular nerve perfusion
A typical hallmark of compression-related neuronal changes is alteration in the nerves microvascular blood supply, which have also been described for CTS.[20–31] In recent years, they have received attention in the sonographic diagnosis of CTS as a semiquantitative criterion of nerve compression (**Fig. 2**).

Nerve Mobility
Compressed nerve structures change their mobility, which can be objectified in both long-axis and short-axis views (Videos 1 and 2). These changes can be dynamically visualized with sonography and evaluated as a semiquantitative feature of compression of the median nerve in the carpal tunnel (Videos 3 and 4).[32–38] They are also relevant to the postoperative assessment,[39] where they can distinguish well between local (persistent) constrictions and adhesions.

Nerve Environment
Changes in the nerve environment can also have an influence on compression. The lower the elasticity of the environment, the less the nerve can yield to external influences. Ultrasound devices nowadays offer the possibility of elastography to measure this tissue elasticity and can thus semiquantitatively determine the compression effect on the nerve in terms of a color-coded mapping.[40–46]

Echogenicity

Another sonographic criterion for nerve compression is the change in the nerve echotexture.[47,48] Usually, a healthy nerve has a honeycomb-like echotexture resulting from the separation of the hypoechoic fascicles by the hyperechoic perineurium.[48] In case of mechanical compression, an edematous thickening of the hypoechoic fascicles occurs with a simultaneous suppression of the perifascicular parts, which causes transformation

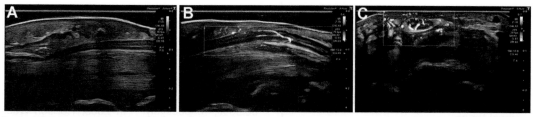

Fig. 2. (*A*) Short-segment compression of the median nerve in the carpal tunnel (long-axis view, B-mode). (*B*) Perineural and epineural hypervascularity of the median nerve at the site of compression (long-axis view, superb microvascular imaging). (*C*) Perineural and epineural hypervascularity of the median nerve at the site of compression (short-axis view, superb microvascular imaging).

of the typical honeycomb structure of the nerve into a predominantly hypoechoic pattern (**Fig. 3**).

Quantitative Criteria of Nerve Compression

Nerve thickness

Because of its possibility of quantitative assessment, thickening of the perineurium and endoneurium and thus of the entire nerve is probably the most relevant criterion of nerve compression on ultrasonography.[19,49–51] Also referred to as pseudoneuroma, it is located prestenotically[19] and can be localized and quantified by imaging techniques such as MRI[52] or sonography.[53] Their extent correlates with the presence of axonal damage.[49]

SONOGRAPHY OF CTS—NOW AND THEN

The sonographic diagnosis of CTS originated from comparative MR examinations between healthy subjects and electrophysiologically verified patients. Mezgarzadeh and colleagues were able to demonstrate typical changes consisting of swelling of the nerve proximal to the carpal tunnel, a flattening in the distal carpal tunnel, and an increased palmar flexion of the transverse carpal ligament.[52,54] They were applied to ultrasonography a few years later[53] and supplemented (**Box 1**).[55]

Preliminary studies focused on the extent of the prestenotic swelling, called pseudoneuroma, which in most publications was assumed to be located at the carpal tunnel entrance. Comparative studies between the pathologically increased CSA in patients with electrophysiologically verified CTS and the CSA of healthy subjects were intended to establish a reference value for the diagnosis of CTS. Comparisons between nerve CSA at the carpal tunnel entrance, which was considered to be located at the pisiform bone, and electrophysiologic parameters were used to determine the severity of the disease, but could hardly meet the expectations, since the cut-offs between 6.5 mm^2 and 15 mm^2 showed a high variability and therefore only a moderate correlation between sonographic and electrophysiologic findings.

The reasons for the poor correlation between nerve conduction studies (NCS) and a single sonographic cut-off value are partly proven and partly speculative:

1. Many of the existing studies are subject to a bias, as electrodiagnostic testing is considered to be the diagnostic gold standard. The patient population filtered in this way also contains false-positive and excludes false-negative cases that might have been negative or positive

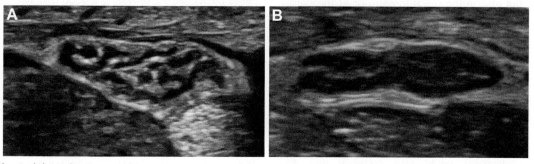

Fig. 3. (*A*) Median nerve (short-axis view, B-mode). Normal honeycomb-like echotexture and echogenicity. (*B*) Median nerve (short-axis view, B-mode). Compression-related hypoechoic alteration of echogenicity and hyperechoic rim (perineurium).

> **Box 1**
> **Sonographic criteria of carpal tunnel syndrome**
>
> *Sonographic Criteria* | Buchberger et al. 1991
>
> Swelling of the median nerve at the entrance of the carpal tunnel
>
> Flattening of the median nerve in the distal carpal tunnel
>
> Increased palmar flexion of the transverse carpal ligament
>
> *Extended Sonographic Criteria* | Buchberger et al. 1992, Beekman et al. 2003
>
> Significant increase in cross-sectional area at the level of the pisiform bone and, to a lesser extent, at the level of the hamate
>
> Significant increase in cross-sectional area at the level of the pisiform bone compared to the cross-sectional area at the level of the distal radius (swelling ratio)
>
> Significant increase in flattening ratio at the level of the hook of the hamate
>
> Significant palmar bowing of the flexor retinaculum

in ultrasound diagnostics. The diagnostic potential of sonography is thereby attenuated. Studies investigating patients with clinical symptoms of CTS and negative NCS seem to better reflect the potential of sonography.[56–61] The same could be assumed for studies using the postoperative outcome as a parameter for the presence of CTS.

2. Apart from methodological differences in study design, different compression levels within the carpal tunnel must be taken into account. Although many studies target the pseudoneuroma at the carpal tunnel inlet, a more proximal or distal compression of the nerve is also possible, as a positive Tinel's sign may be located not only at the carpal tunnel entrance but also in the distal forearm or at the carpal tunnel outlet.

3. The distance between the greatest extent of the nerve swelling and the exact location of the compression, and whether that distance represents a constant, is unclear. It must be assumed that individual factors such as gender,[62,63] origin (**Table 1**), and age[64–67] also play a substantial role. In the same way that age-specific normal values are used in electrodiagnostic testing, the potential to form a pseudoneuroma could also correlate with the patient's age or even with secondary disorders.[68]

Fowler and colleagues performed a meta-analysis comparing the sensitivities and specificities according to different reference standards. Depending on the reference standard used (clinical diagnosis, NCS, and composite), the sensitivities and specificities ranged between 77.3%, 80.2%, and 77.6%, and 92.8%, 78.7%, and 86.85%, respectively.[69] In 2008, Hobson-Webb et al. proposed the use of a wrist-to-forearm ratio, reflecting a comparison of the prestenotic swelling at the level of the wrist and a proximal reference value at the level of the forearm.[70] This method has become widely accepted and has also been used with other locations for reference values (**Table 2**).[71–73] From the authors' point of view, this procedure is recommended to be used in addition to a single cut-off value, especially if there are borderline findings in CSA at the level of the pseudoneuroma. The use of a ratio can increase the sensitivity to values between 93.5% and 99% with a specificity of up to 100%.[71,74] Furthermore, this strategy allows the identification of other pathologies such as multifocal acquired demyelinating sensory and motor neuropathy (MADSAM) (**Fig. 4**).

TECHNICAL ASPECTS AND ULTRASOUND EXAMINATION

Sonographic examination of the median nerve is usually performed on a seated patient. The wrist is placed in a neutral position on a flat surface with the digits semiextended.[75] Sometimes it can be helpful to support the wrist to bring it into a slight hyperextension. Passive traction on the slightly flexed digits can then be applied to check the mobility of the median nerve, which is an important diagnostic criterion, especially in the postoperative situation.

A linear array ultrasound probe with a sonic frequency of 15 to 18 MHz or higher is recommended (**Fig. 5**). In contrast to smaller hockey-stick transducers, it allows the entire width of the carpal tunnel to be visualized, providing a good overview of additional masses or other pathologies. Hockey-stick transducers can be helpful in assessing cubital tunnel syndrome as the winding course of the ulnar nerve at the level of the ulnar condyle can be visualized without any gaps. In contrast, the hockey-stick transducer is usually too small when it comes to visualization of the carpal tunnel in its entire width.

Assessment of the Cut-off Value

The median nerve can be easily located and measured at the carpal tunnel entrance using the specified anatomic landmarks, the pisiform bone,

Table 1
Nerve cross-sectional values of the median nerve in relation to the patient's origin (Schelle 2015)

Author	CSA (mm^2) Mean ± SD	CSA (mm^2) Upper Threshold	Population
Boehm et al. 2014	8.5 ± 1.8	10.3	Europe (Germany, Hungary)
Burg et al. 2014	8.3 ± 1.9	10.2	Europe (The Netherlands)
Tagliafico et al. 2013	8.2 ± 2.3	10.5	Europe (Italy)
Zaidman et al. 2009	9.7 ± 1.9	11.6	North America (USA)
Burg et al. 2014	7.0 ± 1.1	8.1	Asia (India)
Wanitwattanarumlug et al. 2012	6.8 ± 0.9	7.7	Asia (Thailand)
Kim et al. 2014	7.9 ± 1.3	9.2	Asia (Korea)
Azami et al. 2014	8.5 ± 0.8	9.3	Asia (Iran)

and the scaphoid tubercle. For this purpose, the 2 carpal bones are adjusted in short-axis-view and the nerve CSA is measured by direct tracing using the device software (**Fig. 6**). The hyperechoic rim of the nerve should be excluded from the measurement. One reason for this is that the echogenicity of the nerve fascicles is reduced and therefore can be better demarcated from the hyperechoic perineurium than the perineurium from the also hyperechoic connective tissue.

Second, the compression-induced swelling seems to affect the nerve fascicles rather than the perineurium.[76] Especially in cases of a thin perineurium, differentiation of the hypoechoic nerve can be difficult, as the flexor tendons run obliquely relative to the surface and therefore are subject to the artifact of anisotropy, which causes them to appear hypoechoic as well. If this is the case, it might be helpful to tilt the transducer slightly to distal (Video 5) or to trace the nerve proximally

Table 2
Selected diagnostic parameters of carpal tunnel syndrome

Level I Evidence Studies		
CSA $_{Wrist\ Level}$ (cut-off) $\geq$ 0.085 cm^2	Sensitivity 97% | Specificity 98%	Mohammadi et al. 2010
CSA $_{Wrist\ Level}$ (cut-off) $\geq$ 0.10 cm^2	Sensitivity 82% | Specificity 87%	Ziswiler et al. 2005
CSA $_{Wrist-to-Forearm\ Ratio}$ $\geq$ 1.4	Sensitivity 100%	Hobson-Webb et al. 2008
CSA $_{Wrist\ Level}$ + CSA $_{Wrist-to-Forearm\ Ratio}$ $\geq$ 1.4		Billakota et al. 2017
Meta-Analyses		
28 Studies | 3995 Extremities	Sensitivity 87% | Specificity 83% for CSA $_{Wrist\ Level}$ $\geq$ 0.09 cm^2	Tai et al. 2012
13 Studies	Sensitivity 84% | Specificity 74% (pooled) for CSA $_{Wrist\ Level}$ $\geq$ 9.5–10.5 mm^2	Descata et al. 2012
Bifid Median Nerve (Level II Evidence Studies)		
CSA $_{Wrist\ Level}$ (cut-off) $\geq$ 0.12 cm^2	Sensitivity 85% | Specificity 47%	Klauser et al. 2001
CSA $_{Wrist\ Level}$ − CSA $_{Forearm}$ $\geq$ 4 mm^2	Sensitivity 93% | Specificity 95%	

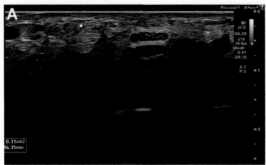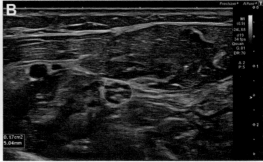

Fig. 4. (*A*) and (*B*) Median nerve (short-axis view, B-mode) showing slight increase in nerve CSA at the carpal tunnel entrance (11 mm^2) and fascicular hypertrophy at forearm level (17mm^2) indicating multifocal acquired demyelinating sensory and motor neuropathy (MADSAM).

by short-axis sliding up to the point where the honeycomb echotexture becomes visible again. A higher reliability to identify the pseudoneuroma at its proper localization is given if the nerve is visualized in long-axis view. The full extent of compression is then typically seen as an hourglass-shaped constriction under the flexorum retinaculum with the pseudoneuroma located proximal to it (**Fig. 7**). The CSA can then be measured individually after rotating the transducer by 90°. This technique gives a complete overview of the entire course of the median nerve throughout the carpal tunnel and even ensures the localization of a pseudoneuroma in the distal part of the carpal tunnel or at the carpal tunnel outlet (**Fig. 8**). If necessary, the median nerve can also be traced in the long-axis view (Video 6). If ultrasound assessment reveals a high division of the nerve or a bifid median nerve, the CSA can also be determined. In these cases, the nerve cross-sectional areas of both nerve portions are simply added together (**Fig. 9**).[77]

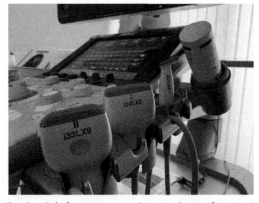

Fig. 5. High-frequency matrix transducers for use in nerve sonography. Although sound frequencies between 15 and 24 MHz provide an optimal balance between resolution and penetration depth, higher frequencies (eg, 33 MHz) can increase resolution and diagnostic accuracy in the imaging of superficial sensory cutaneous nerves or pediatric patients.

Determining a Reference Value

The relationship of cut-off value to a reference is calculated using either a swelling ratio or a flattening ratio (**Fig. 10**). To determine the swelling ratio, the measurement of a proximal reference value is required, which is also obtained in the short-axis view. Starting from the cut-off value at the level of the pseudoneuroma, the desired proximal reference point can be reached by short-axis sliding (Video 7) and the CSA can be determined by direct tracing as well (**Fig. 11**). Determining the change in relationship between proximal reference value and pseudoneuroma (swelling ratio) leads to an increase in the sensitivity of sonographic diagnosis of CTS.[73]

Diagnosis of CTS can be alternatively (or supplementary) made by determining a flattening ratio.[73,74,78–82] In contrast to the swelling ratio, the pseudoneuroma is here related to the distal flattening of the nerve. In the authors' view, this procedure is more difficult to reproduce as the median nerve is increasingly subject to the artifact of anisotropy in its distal course and is more difficult to define in cross-section. This is further aggravated by the fact that the median nerve may have already divided at this level. All in all, however, the supplementary measurement of the CSA at the level of the carpal tunnel outlet seems to provide a further increase in sensitivity.[80,82] Olde Dubbelink and colleagues describe a completely different approach in which the nerve cross-sectional area is related to the circumference of the wrist.[83]

RATING SONOGRAPHIC DIAGNOSTICS
Exclusion Diagnostics

With high-resolution ultrasound, the diagnosis of CTS has been improved by a very valuable procedure. Using a sonographic ratio between prestenotic swelling and ipsilateral comparative

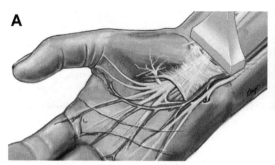

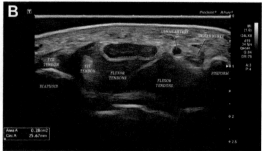

Fig. 6. (A) Placement of the transducer at the carpal tunnel entrance to determine the CSA of the pseudoneuroma. (B) Median nerve (short-axis view, B-mode) at the carpal tunnel entrance defined by the bony landmarks of the scaphoid and pisiform bones. Hypoechoic appearance of the flexor tendons due to the artifact of anisotropy.

value or a flattening ratio, ultrasound provides a reliable exclusion diagnosis of the disease without the need for additional NCS. At the same time, however, sonography is a useful complementary procedure to electrodiagnostic testing.[84] Especially in cases where typical symptoms and clinical parameters of CTS are present and cannot be confirmed by NCS, ultrasonography can help to establish the diagnosis.[56–61] If both NCS and sonography are negative, steroid infiltration may be considered as an additional diagnostic tool. Its ultrasound-guided application has additional advantages over a blind, landmark-associated approach (**Fig. 12**).[85,86]

Disease Severity

In CTS (and other compression neuropathies), preoperative assessment of disease severity provides an individual impression of the necessity and urgency of surgical treatment and draws an imaginary picture of the existing nerve damage. In contrast to NCS, in which the signal is recorded over a defined segment including the localization of the compression, the shape and the amount of the pseudoneuroma relevant for sonographic diagnosis varies from individual to individual.

Furthermore, its localization is not precisely defined anatomically. A direct comparison of both methods is therefore only possible to a limited extent. Electrodiagnostic parameters such as distal motor latency, nerve conduction velocity, and others allow sufficient quantification of the disease. Although a correlation between nerve cross-sectional area and electrodiagnostic parameters has been clearly demonstrated,[87] the correlation coefficients of most comparative studies are only moderate. Therefore, statements about disease severity after sonographic diagnosis alone are not possible or should be regarded with caution.[84,88,89] In the assessment of disease severity, ultrasonography is therefore only a complementary additional diagnostic tool to NCS, which at best allows orienting statements on disease severity and, with regard to postoperative nerve regeneration and sufficiency of nerve decompression, does not reach the accuracy of NCS.

Causes of Nerve Compression

In addition to the possibility of a reliable exclusion diagnosis, ultrasound examination has further advantages for patients and therapists, as important

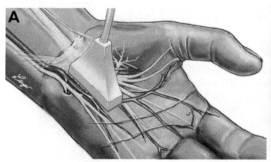

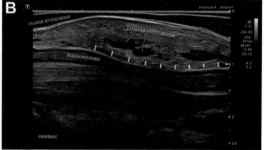

Fig. 7. (A) Positioning of the transducer along the median nerve for proper localization of the pseudoneuroma. (B) Median nerve (long-axis view, B-mode) at the level of the carpal tunnel for proper localization of the pseudoneuroma, just proximal to the flexor retinaculum (*white arrows*).

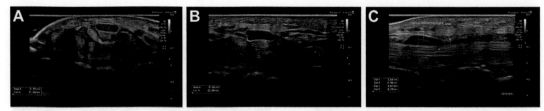

Fig. 8. (*A*) Median nerve (short-axis view, B-mode) at the carpal tunnel entrance. Extensive synovitis of the flexor tendons with increase in nerve cross-sectional area to 15 mm^2. (*B*) Median nerve (short-axis view, B-mode) at the carpal tunnel outlet. In addition to the pseudoneuroma at the carpal tunnel entrance, a distal pseudoneuroma with a nerve cross-sectional area of 24 mm^2 can be identified. (*C*) Median nerve (long-axis view, B-mode) at the middle and distal aspects of the carpal tunnel. The long-axis view provides additional information on the pseudoneuroma at the carpal tunnel outlet.

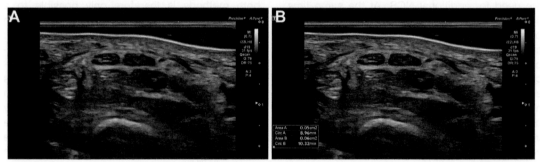

Fig. 9. (*A*) Bifid median nerve (short-axis view, B-mode) at the carpal tunnel entrance. (*B*). Bifid median nerve (short-axis view, B-mode) at the carpal tunnel entrance. Separate direct tracing of the 2 nerve segments.

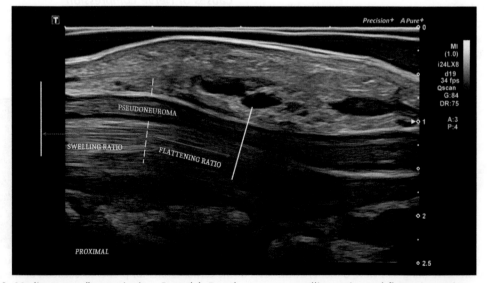

Fig. 10. Median nerve (long-axis view, B-mode). Pseudoneuroma, swelling ratio, and flattening ratio.

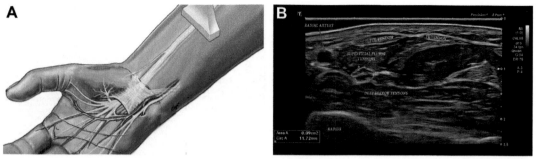

Fig. 11. (A) Transducer positioning approximately 12 cm proximal to the distal wrist crease to determine the reference value according to Hobson-Webb et al. (see also **Table 2**). (B). Median nerve (short-axis view, B-mode). Transducer positioning approximately 12 cm proximal to the distal wrist crease and measurement of the nerve cross-sectional area by direct tracing.

additional information can be obtained. Atypical findings and causes of compression such as marked synovitis,[90] hypertrophic or aberrant muscle fibers,[91] nerve subluxations,[92] intraneural space-occupying lesions,[93] a high division of the median nerve, variant branches and isolated compressions of the thenar motor branch (**Fig. 13**),[94] a bifid median nerve with a median artery (**Fig. 14**),[77,95–104] trifid nerves[105] but also compressing wrist ganglion cysts (**Fig. 15**) or crystal deposition diseases (**Fig. 16**), nerve[106] and tendon sheath tumors (**Fig. 17**) can be identified and will guide the surgical approach. Dynamic assessments facilitate the diagnosis of dynamic compressions as they occur in postoperative

adhesions (Video 8)[107,108] but also in muscle variants (**Fig. 18**) (Videos 9 and 10),[91,109] and anomalous tendon slips[110] and may be induced by certain activities.[111] In addition, sonography allows for sonographically guided infiltrations and therapies with a proven lower complication rate than a blind approach.[85,86]

Postoperative Diagnostics

A quantitative assessment is not only of preoperative interest. Quantitative parameters are also of prognostic relevance in the event of no improvement in postoperative findings. The direct comparison between the preoperative and postoperative

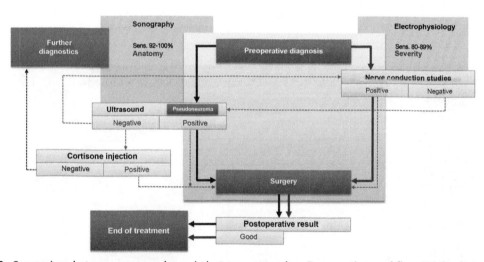

Fig. 12. Comparison between sonography and electroneurography—Preoperative workflow. While electrodiagnostic testing can diagnose carpal tunnel syndrome with a sensitivity of 80% to 89%, the sensitivity of sonography is about 92% to 100%. Electrodiagnostic testing basically allows statements to be made about the severity of the disease (*right*), whereas sonography focuses primarily on quantitative and semiquantitative parameters (*left*). In the case of negative findings in either electrophysiology or sonography, both examination modalities can complement each other. In the case of negative findings on both sides, diagnostic steroid infiltration can help to confirm the diagnosis, which is also possible under sonographic guidance.

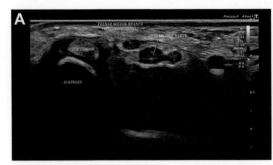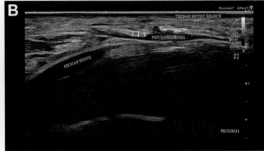

Fig. 13. (*A*) Bifid median nerve (short-axis view, B-mode) at the carpal tunnel entrance. Anatomic variant and isolated compression and pseudoneuroma of the thenar motor branch along its path throughout the flexor retinaculum. (*B*). Thenar motor branch of the median nerve (long-axis view, B-mode) along its path throughout the flexor retinaculum with isolated compression (*white arrows*) and visible pseudoneuroma formation.

situation requires parameters that correlate as closely as possible with the severity of the disease preoperatively and with the improvement in findings postoperatively. Unfortunately, scientific interest has been predominantly focused on preoperative diagnostics, which is why a limited number of studies, at best, have addressed sonography of CTS in preoperative and postoperative comparisons.[112–123]

In addition to the previously mentioned limited correlation of quantitative values of preoperative sonography and NCS, the sonographic quantification of the disease also appears to be limited postoperatively.[114,116,119,124] Although clinical improvement is associated with regression of the CSA,[113,115,119,120] this turns out to be much slower in direct comparison to normalization of electrodiagnostic values.[117–119,121] Temporarily, there is even an increase in nerve CSA at the level of the carpal tunnel outlet postoperatively.[120] Even the wrist-to-forearm ratio seems to have no further benefit here,[122] and it may even be possible that residual swelling must be assumed in the long term.[117,121]

From the authors' point of view, several postoperative situations have to be covered, which can basically be classified into 3 main scenarios, each of them requiring an individually adapted additional diagnostic approach:

- The probably most frequent situation is the one in which subjectively no postoperative improvement of findings occurs even after a considerable waiting period. In the case of severe CTS, this is quite common, but occasionally causes operatively treated patients to question the success of the surgery. In this

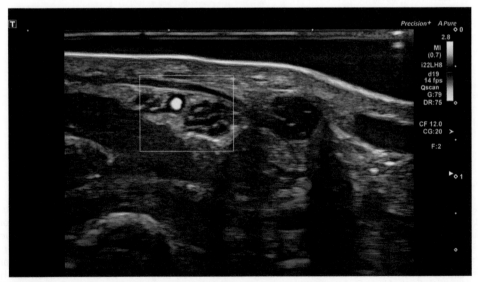

Fig. 14. Bifid median nerve with median artery (short-axis view, B-mode).

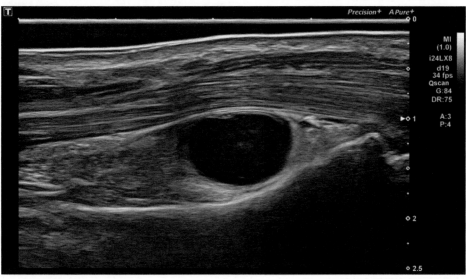

Fig. 15. Large palmar wrist ganglion cyst in the pronator quadratus muscle with compression of the median nerve (long-axis view, B-mode).

case, improvement in short-term follow-up is most accurately demonstrated by NCS, which is only possible if preoperative baseline values exist. Although electrophysiologic parameters do not linearly correlate with the extent of clinical improvement,[125] NCS still allow a more reliable and accurate monitoring in short-term follow-up compared to sonography. In contrast, normalization of the sonographically determined CSA appears to occur much more slowly,[117–120,122] indicating that sonography is

less suitable for an early postoperative follow-up assessment.
- The situation is different, in patients who tend to complain of an increase in symptoms postoperatively. In this case, incomplete decompression (unrelieved CTS)[126,127] or even a nerve injury must be assumed, which are easy to differentiate sonographically. While in the case of a nerve injury, a discontinuity of the nerve structure or partial disruption of the perineurium can be visualized (**Fig. 19**), persistent compression usually results in a

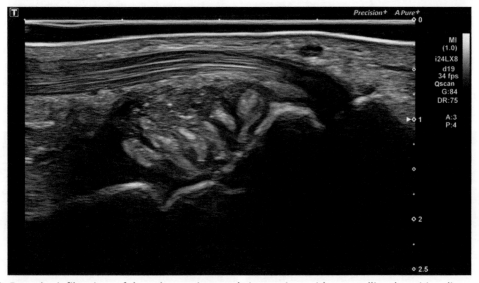

Fig. 16. Extensive infiltrations of the palmar wrist capsule in a patient with a crystalline deposition disease. Kinking and compression of the median nerve (long-axis view, B-mode).

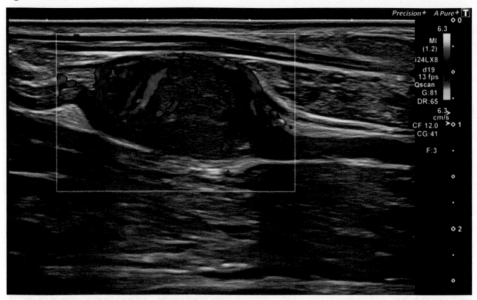

Fig. 17. Median nerve proximal to the carpal tunnel inlet (long-axis view, Doppler-mode). Nerve sheath tumor (Schwannoma) with typical hypervascularity.

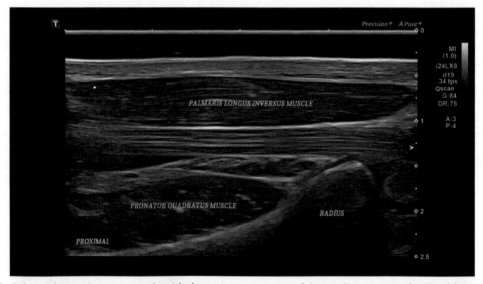

Fig. 18. Palmaris longus inversus muscle with dynamic compression of the median nerve at the distal forearm/carpal tunnel inlet (long-axis view, B-mode).

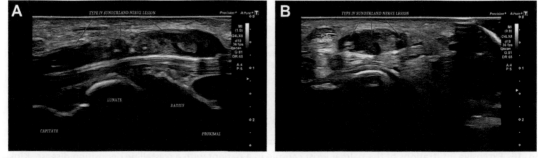

Fig. 19. (*A*) Median nerve (long-axis view, B-mode). Type IV Sunderland nerve lesion with neuroma in continuity after endoscopic carpal tunnel release. (*B*) Median nerve (short-axis view, B-mode). Type IV Sunderland nerve lesion with neuroma in continuity after endoscopic carpal tunnel release.

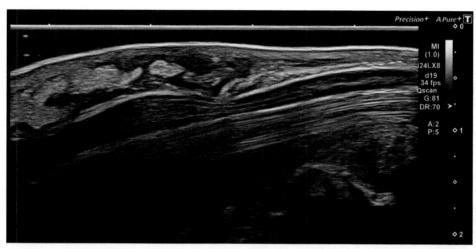

Fig. 20. Median nerve at the carpal tunnel (long-axis view, B-mode). Persistent short-segment compression of the median nerve after surgical treatment of carpal tunnel syndrome.

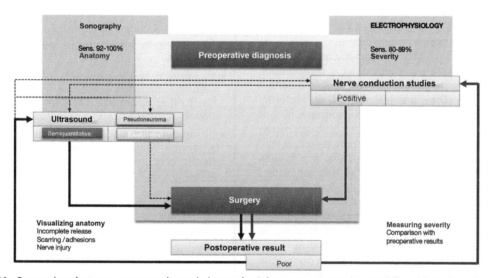

Fig. 21. Comparison between sonography and electrophysiology—postoperative workflow. The value of postoperative ultrasound lies in the visualization of the anatomy. While preoperative ultrasound diagnostics focus on the CSA of the median nerve, in the postoperative setting mainly semiquantitative sonographic parameters such as mobility and scarring are of interest. NCS, on the other side, provide a direct comparison of preoperative and postoperative nerve function if preoperative baseline values have been obtained. Depending on the specific postoperative situation, both diagnostic modalities have their specific indications and can complement each other.

short-segment stenosis, which can best be localized in the long-axis view (**Fig. 20**). Because of the overall decompression of the nerve, an increase of the pseudoneuroma is recognizable,[108] which can be quantified in the short-axis view. In contrast, NCS are less relevant in the first 14 to 21 days and have only supplementary value in the long term. The same applies to symptoms of a CTS after previous surgical treatment of a radius fracture, which are a primary indication for ultrasound diagnostics, especially since the severity of CTS plays a secondary role in this specific situation. Pre-existing symptoms and those exacerbated by the surgical procedure can be diagnosed based on the pseudoneuroma. Irritation of the nerve by the access trauma should also be taken into account. It is usually the result of an incorrectly performed Henry approach in which the radius is not approached radial to the FCR tendon but ulnarly between the FCR tendon and the median nerve. In these cases, adhesions of the median nerve are frequently observed along the surgical approach, which can be visualized in short-axis view proximal to the carpal tunnel inlet. Dynamic assessment with active flexion of the digits usually confirms adhesions of the nerve to the muscle fibers of the long finger flexors. Lacerations of the median nerve are also visible as loss of continuity. Lesions of the palmar branch of the median nerve can be visualized as a loss of continuity in the early course, later by visualizing a hypoechoic neuroma.

• The third situation describes cases in which the symptoms of median nerve compression improve initially but reappear after a certain period. They are referred to as recurrent CTS. Whether a complete normalization of the nerve CSA or the swelling ratio can be expected and when it will occur remains unclear. It rather must be assumed that the median nerve is subject to a certain memory effect with persistent residual swelling.[121] Ultrasound diagnostics in this situation is therefore focused on the semiquantitative parameters mentioned above, primarily on changes in gliding behavior and postoperative scarring.[107,108] This should be done in correlation with electrodiagnostic testing which, in some degree, allows a differentiation between persistent and residual changes. The value of postoperative ultrasound lies in the visualization of the anatomy and the conclusions that can be drawn from it.[107,128] It focuses primarily on the semiquantitative sonographic parameters of nerve compression such as mobility,[129,130] postoperative adhesions, and scarring.[107,108] Postoperative ultrasound is mainly based on the causes of persistent complaints rather than quantifying the CSA, which was focused on preoperatively.[131] Nerve lesions as well as persistent strictures can be visualized[126,127,131–133] and clearly localized, especially in the long-axis view. Imaging of postoperative subluxations[92] and compressive hematoma formations is also straightforward. In recurrent disease, the primary focus is to dynamically exclude postoperative scarring, which results in a reduction of nerve gliding (**Fig. 21**).[134]

CLINICS CARE POINTS

- Electrodiagnostic testing still represents the gold standard in confirmatory diagnostics of carpal tunnel syndrome. It allows sufficient quantification of the disease and the reliable differentiation from other compressions of the median nerve.

- US provides a reliable exclusion diagnosis of the disease without the need for additional NCS and is a useful complementary procedure to electrodiagnostic testing.

- In cases where typical symptoms of CTS are present and cannot be confirmed by NCS, ultrasonography can help to establish the diagnosis.

- In addition to the possibility of a reliable exclusion diagnosis, ultrasound examination has further advantages, as important additional information can be obtained.

- Ultrasonografic diagnosis of carpal tunnel syndrome is based on changes in nerve perfusion, nerve mobility, nerve environment, echogenicity, and nerve thickness.

- Preoperative sonographic examination mainly focuses on the pathologically increased CSA of the median nerve proximal to the compression site (pseudoneuroma).

- In the assessment of disease severity, ultrasonography is only a complementary additional diagnostic tool to NCS, which at best allows orienting statements on disease severity and, with regard to postoperative nerve regeneration, does not reach the accuracy of NCS. Statements about disease severity after sonographic diagnosis alone should be regarded with caution.

- Determining the change in relationship between a reference value and pseudoneuroma (swelling ratio / flattening ratio) leads to an increase in the sensitivity of sonographic diagnosis of CTS.
- The use of a ratio between a proximal or distal reference value in addition to a single cut-off value can increase the sensitivity to values between 93.5% and 99% and a specifici

SUPPLEMENTARY DATA

Supplementary data related to this article can be found online at https://doi.org/10.1016/j.hcl.2021.08.003.

REFERENCES

1. Atroshi I, Gummesson C, Johnsson R, et al. Prevalence of carpal tunnel syndrome in a general population. Jama 1999;282(2):153–8.
2. Bland JDP. Carpal tunnel syndrome. Curr Opin Neurol 2005;18(5):581–5.
3. Dyck P, Low PA, C SJ. Diseases of peripheral nerves. In: Backer AB, editor. Clinical Neurology. 1st edition. Philadelphia: Harper and Row; 1985. p. 41–3.
4. Phalen GS, Gardner WJ, La Londe AA. Neuropathy of the median nerve due to compression beneath the transverse carpal ligament. J Bone Joint Surg Am 1950;32A(1):109–12.
5. Sarria L, Cabada T, Cozcolluela R, et al. Carpal tunnel syndrome: usefulness of sonography [review]. Eur Radiol 2000;10:1920–5.
6. Bleecker ML, Bohlman M, Moreland R, et al. Carpal tunnel syndrome: role of carpal canal size. Neurology 1985;35(11):1599–604.
7. Johnson EW, Gatens T, Poindexter D, et al. Wrist dimensions: correlation with median sensory latencies. Arch Phys Med Rehabil 1983;64(11):556–7.
8. Kamolz L-P, Beck H, Haslik W, et al. Carpal tunnel syndrome: a question of hand and wrist configurations? J Hand Surg Eur 2004;29(4):321–4. https://doi.org/10.1016/j.jhsb.2003.09.010.
9. Shiri R. A square-shaped wrist as a predictor of carpal tunnel syndrome: a meta-analysis. Muscle Nerve 2015;52(5):709–13. https://doi.org/10.1002/mus.24761.
10. Tabatabaeifar S, Svendsen SW, Johnsen B, et al. Reversible median nerve impairment after three weeks of repetitive work. Scand J Work Environ Health 2017;43(2):163–70.
11. Bueno-Gracia E, Ruiz de Escudero-Zapico A, Malo-Urries M, et al. Dimensional changes of the carpal tunnel and the median nerve during manual mobilization of the carpal bones. Musculoskelet Sci Pract 2018;36:12–6.
12. Werthel J-D, Zhao C, An K-N, et al. Carpal tunnel syndrome pathophysiology: role of subsynovial connective tissue. Jnl Wrist Surg 2014;03(04):220–6.
13. Festen-Schrier VJMM, Amadio PC. The biomechanics of subsynovial connective tissue in health and its role in carpal tunnel syndrome. J Electromyogr Kinesiol 2018;38:232–9.
14. Cate Ten DF, Glaser N, Luime JJ, et al. A comparison between ultrasonographic, surgical and histological assessment of tenosynovits in a cohort of idiopathic carpal tunnel syndrome patients. Clin Rheumatol 2016;35(3):775–80.
15. Tat J, Wilson KE, Keir PJ. Pathological changes in the subsynovial connective tissue increase with self-reported carpal tunnel syndrome symptoms. Clin Biomech (Bristol, Avon) 2015;30(4):360–5.
16. Graham B. The value added by electrodiagnostic testing in the diagnosis of carpal tunnel syndrome. J Bone Joint Surg Am 2008;90(12):2587–93.
17. American Association of Electrodiagnostic Medicine, American Academy of Neurology, and American Academy of Physical Medicine and Rehabilitation. Practice parameter for electrodiagnostic studies in carpal tunnel syndrome: summary statement. Muscle Nerve 2002;25(6):918–22.
18. Löscher WN, Auer-Grumbach M, Trinka E, et al. Comparison of second lumbrical and interosseus latencies with standard measures of median nerve function across the carpal tunnel: a prospective study of 450 hands. J Neurol 2000;247(7):530–4.
19. Rempel D, Dahlin L, Lundborg G. Pathophysiology of nerve compression syndromes: response of peripheral nerves to loading. J Bone Joint Surg Am 1999;81(11):1600–10.
20. Dejaco C, Stradner M, Zauner D, et al. Ultrasound for diagnosis of carpal tunnel syndrome: comparison of different methods to determine median nerve volume and value of power Doppler sonography. Ann Rheum Dis 2012;72(12):1934–9.
21. Ghasemi-Esfe AR, Khalilzadeh O, Mazloumi M, et al. Combination of high-resolution and color Doppler ultrasound in diagnosis of carpal tunnel syndrome. Acta Radiol 2011;52(2):191–7.
22. Ghasemi-Esfe AR, Khalilzadeh O, Vaziri-Bozorg SM, et al. Color and power Doppler US for diagnosing carpal tunnel syndrome and determining its severity: a quantitative image processing method. Radiology 2011;261(2):499–506.
23. Ghasemi-Esfe AR, Morteza A, Khalilzadeh O, et al. Color Doppler ultrasound for evaluation of vasomotor activity in patients with carpal tunnel syndrome. Skeletal Radiol 2012;41(3):281–6.
24. Joy V, Therimadasamy AK, Chan YC, et al. Combined Doppler and B-mode sonography in carpal

tunnel syndrome. J Neurol Sci 2011;308(1–2): 16–20.

25. Kutlar N, Bayrak AO, Bayrak İK, et al. Diagnosing carpal tunnel syndrome with Doppler ultrasonography: a comparison of ultrasonographic measurements and electrophysiological severity. Neurol Res 2017;39(2):126–32.

26. Mallouhi A, Pülzl P, Pültzl P, et al. Predictors of carpal tunnel syndrome: accuracy of gray-scale and color Doppler sonography. AJR Am J Roentgenol 2006;186(5):1240–5.

27. Mohammadi A, Ghasemi-Rad M, Mladkova-Suchy N, et al. Correlation between the severity of carpal tunnel syndrome and color Doppler sonography findings. AJR Am J Roentgenol 2012; 198(2):W181–4.

28. Motomiya M, Funakoshi T, Iwasaki N. Intraneural microvascular patterns of the median nerve assessed using contrast-enhanced ultrasonography in carpal tunnel syndrome. J Hand Surg Eur 2015; 41(2). 1753193415570222-1753193415570231.

29. Ng ES, Ng KW, Wilder-Smith EP. Provocation tests in doppler ultrasonography for carpal tunnel syndrome. Muscle Nerve 2013;47(1):116–7.

30. Karahan AY, Arslan S, Ordahan B, et al. Superb microvascular imaging of the median nerve in carpal tunnel syndrome: an electrodiagnostic and ultrasonographic study. J Ultrasound Med 2018;94: 45.

31. Chen J, Chen L, Wu L, et al. Value of superb microvascular imaging ultrasonography in the diagnosis of carpal tunnel syndrome: Compared with color Doppler and power Doppler. Medicine (Baltimore) 2017;96(21):e6862.

32. Wang Y, Filius A, Zhao C, et al. Altered median nerve deformation and transverse displacement during wrist movement in patients with carpal tunnel syndrome. Acad Radiol 2014;21(4):472–80.

33. Liong K, Lahiri A, Lee S, et al. Predominant patterns of median nerve displacement and deformation during individual finger motion in early carpal tunnel syndrome. Ultrasound Med Biol 2014; 40(8):1810–8.

34. Kang HJ, Yoon JS. Effect of finger motion on transverse median nerve movement in the carpal tunnel. Muscle Nerve 2016;54(4):738–42.

35. Ellis R, Blyth R, Arnold N, et al. Is there a relationship between impaired median nerve excursion and carpal tunnel syndrome? A systematic review. J Hand Ther 2016;0(0).

36. Kuo T-T, Lee M-R, Liao Y-Y, et al. Assessment of median nerve mobility by ultrasound dynamic imaging for diagnosing carpal tunnel syndrome. PLoS ONE 2016;11:e0147051.

37. Park D. Ultrasonography of the transverse movement and deformation of the median nerve and its relationships with electrophysiological severity in the early stages of carpal tunnel syndrome. PM R 2017;9(11):1085–94.

38. Park G-Y, Kwon DR, Seok JI, et al. Usefulness of ultrasound assessment of median nerve mobility in carpal tunnel syndrome. Acta Radiol 2018;139. 284185118762246.

39. Schrier VJMM, Evers S, Geske JR, et al. Median nerve transverse mobility and outcome after carpal tunnel release. Ultrasound Med Biol 2019;45(11):2887–97.

40. Miyamoto H, Morizaki Y, Kashiyama T, et al. Grey-scale sonography and sonoelastography for diagnosing carpal tunnel syndrome. World J Radiol 2016;8(3):281–7.

41. Cingoz M, Kandemirli SG, Alis DC, et al. Evaluation of median nerve by shear wave elastography and diffusion tensor imaging in carpal tunnel syndrome. Eur J Radiol 2018;101:59–64.

42. Arslan H, Yavuz A, İlgen F, et al. The efficiency of acoustic radiation force impulse (ARFI) elastography in the diagnosis and staging of carpal tunnel syndrome. J Med Ultrason (2001) 2018;14(3):29–37.

43. Kubo K, Zhou B, Cheng Y-S, et al. Ultrasound elastography for carpal tunnel pressure measurement: A cadaveric validation study. J Orthop Res 2018; 36(1):477–83.

44. Wee TC, Simon NG. Ultrasound elastography for the evaluation of peripheral nerves - A systematic review. Muscle Nerve 2019;60(5):26624–7512.

45. Ghajarzadeh M, Dadgostar M, Sarraf P, et al. Application of ultrasound elastography for determining carpal tunnel syndrome severity. Jpn J Radiol 2015;33(5):273–8.

46. Klauser AS, Miyamoto H, Martinoli C, et al. Sonoelastographic findings of carpal tunnel injection. Ultraschall Med 2015;36(6):618–22.

47. Wilder-Smith EP. Quantitative assessment of peripheral nerve ultrasound echogenicity. A step forward. Clin Neurophysiol 2012;123(7):1267–8.

48. Tagliafico A, Tagliafico G, Martinoli C. Nerve density: a new parameter to evaluate peripheral nerve pathology on ultrasound. Preliminary study. Ultrasound Med Biol 2010;36(10):1588–93.

49. Beekman R, Visser LH. Sonography in the diagnosis of carpal tunnel syndrome: a critical review of the literature. Muscle Nerve 2003;27(1):26–33.

50. Dahlin LB, Lundborg G. The neurone and its response to peripheral nerve compression. J Hand Surg Br 1990;15(1):5–10.

51. Lundborg G, Dahlin LB. Anatomy, function, and pathophysiology of peripheral nerves and nerve compression. Hand Clin 1996;12(2):185–93.

52. Mesgarzadeh M, Schneck CD, Bonakdarpour A, et al. Carpal tunnel: MR imaging. Part II. Carpal tunnel syndrome. Radiology 1989;171(3):749–54.

53. Buchberger W, Schön G, Strasser K, et al. High-resolution ultrasonography of the carpal tunnel. J Ultrasound Med 1991;10(10):531–7.

54. Mesgarzadeh M, Schneck CD, Bonakdarpour A. Carpal tunnel: MR imaging. Part I. Normal anatomy. Radiology 1989;171(3):743–8.

55. Buchberger W, Judmaier W, Birbamer G, et al. Carpal tunnel syndrome: diagnosis with high-resolution sonography. AJR Am J Roentgenol 1992;159(4):793–8.

56. Koyuncuoglu HR, Kutluhan S, Yesildag A, et al. The value of ultrasonographic measurement in carpal tunnel syndrome in patients with negative electrodiagnostic tests. Eur J Radiol 2005;56(3):365–9.

57. Al-Hashel JY, Rashad HM, Nouh MR, et al. Sonography in carpal tunnel syndrome with normal nerve conduction studies. Muscle Nerve 2015;51(4):592–7.

58. Borire AA, Hughes AR, Lueck CJ, et al. Sonographic differences in carpal tunnel syndrome with normal and abnormal nerve conduction studies. J Clin Neurosci 2016;34:77–80.

59. Aseem F, Williams JW, Walker FO, et al. Neuromuscular ultrasound in patients with carpal tunnel syndrome and normal nerve conduction studies. Muscle Nerve 2016;39(suppl):495.

60. Aktürk S, Büyükavcı R, Ersoy Y. Median nerve ultrasound in carpal tunnel syndrome with normal electrodiagnostic tests. Acta Neurol Belg 2018;6:69–75.

61. Roghani RS, Holisaz MT, Norouzi AAS, et al. Sensitivity of high-resolution ultrasonography in clinically diagnosed carpal tunnel syndrome patients with hand pain and normal nerve conduction studies. J Pain Res 2018;11:1319–25.

62. Lakshminarayanan K, Shah R, Li Z-M. Sex-related differences in carpal arch morphology. In: Araújo GCS de, editor. PLoS ONE 2019;14(5):e0217425.

63. Gruber L, Gruber H, Djurdjevic T, et al. Gender influence on clinical presentation and high-resolution ultrasound findings in primary carpal tunnel syndrome: do women only differ in incidence? J Med Ultrason (2001) 2016;43(3):413–20.

64. Altinok T, Karakas HM. Ultrasonographic evaluation of age-related changes in bowing of the flexor retinaculum. Surg Radiol Anat 2004;26(6):501–3.

65. Miwa T, Miwa H. Ultrasonography of carpal tunnel syndrome: clinical significance and limitations in elderly patients. Intern Med 2011;50(19):2157–61.

66. Nkrumah G, Blackburn AR, Goitz RJ, et al. Ultrasonography findings in severe carpal tunnel syndrome. Hand (N Y) 2018;77(1). 1558944718788642.

67. Li X, Li JW, Ho AM-H, et al. Age-related differences in the quantitative echo texture of the median nerve. J Ultrasound Med 2015;34(5):797–804.

68. Gregoris N, Bland J. Is carpal tunnel syndrome in the elderly a separate entity? Evidence from median nerve ultrasound. Muscle Nerve 2019;60(3):217–8.

69. Fowler JR, Gaughan JP, Ilyas AM. The sensitivity and specificity of ultrasound for the diagnosis of carpal tunnel syndrome: a meta-analysis. Clin Orthop Relat Res 2011;469(4):1089–94.

70. Hobson-Webb LD, Massey JM, Juel VC, et al. The ultrasonographic wrist-to-forearm median nerve area ratio in carpal tunnel syndrome. Clin Neurophysiol 2008;119(6):1353–7.

71. Klauser AS, Halpern EJ, De Zordo T, et al. Carpal tunnel syndrome assessment with US: value of additional cross-sectional area measurements of the median nerve in patients versus healthy volunteers. Radiology 2009;250(1):171–7.

72. Kluge S, Kreutziger J, Hennecke B, et al. Inter- and intraobserver reliability of predefined diagnostic levels in high-resolution sonography of the carpal tunnel syndrome - a validation study on healthy volunteers. Ultraschall Med 2010;31(1):43–7.

73. Lee KM, Kim HJ. Relationship between electrodiagnosis and various ultrasonographic findings for diagnosis of carpal tunnel syndrome. Ann Rehabil Med 2016;40(6):1040–7.

74. Azman D, Hrabač P, Demarin V. Use of multiple ultrasonographic parameters in confirmation of carpal tunnel syndrome. J Ultrasound Med 2018;37(4):879–89.

75. Kuo MH, Leong CP, Cheng YF, et al. Static wrist position associated with least median nerve compression: sonographic evaluation. Am J Phys Med Rehabil 2001;80(4):256–60.

76. Wong SM, Griffith JF, Hui ACF, et al. Discriminatory sonographic criteria for the diagnosis of carpal tunnel syndrome. Arthritis Rheum 2002;46(7):1914–21.

77. Klauser AS, Halpern EJ, Faschingbauer R, et al. Bifid median nerve in carpal tunnel syndrome: assessment with US cross-sectional area measurement. Radiology 2011;259(3):808–15.

78. Wong SM, Griffith JF, Hui ACF, et al. Carpal tunnel syndrome: diagnostic usefulness of sonography. Radiology 2004;232(1):93–9.

79. Moran L, Perez M, Esteban A, et al. Sonographic measurement of cross-sectional area of the median nerve in the diagnosis of carpal tunnel syndrome: correlation with nerve conduction studies. J Clin Ultrasound 2009;37(3):125–31.

80. Paliwal PR, Therimadasamy AK, Chan YC, et al. Does measuring the median nerve at the carpal tunnel outlet improve ultrasound CTS diagnosis? J Neurol Sci 2014;339(1–2):47–51.

81. Fu T, Cao M, Liu F, et al. Carpal tunnel syndrome assessment with ultrasonography: value of inlet-to-outlet median nerve area ratio in patients versus healthy volunteers. In: Stover CM, editor. PLoS ONE 2015;10(1):e0116777.

82. Csillik A, Bereczki D, Bora L, et al. The significance of ultrasonographic carpal tunnel outlet

measurements in the diagnosis of carpal tunnel syndrome. Clin Neurophysiol 2016;127(12): 3516–23.

83. Olde Dubbelink TBG, De Kleermaeker FGCM, Meulstee J, et al. Augmented diagnostic accuracy of ultrasonography for diagnosing carpal tunnel syndrome using an optimised wrist circumference-dependent cross-sectional area equation. Front Neurol 2020;11:577052.

84. Billakota S, Hobson-Webb LD. Standard median nerve ultrasound in carpal tunnel syndrome: a retrospective review of 1,021 cases. Clin Neurophysiol Pract 2017;2:188–91.

85. Chen P-C, Wang L-Y, Pong Y-P, et al. Effectiveness of ultrasound-guided vs direct approach corticosteroid injections for carpal tunnel syndrome: a double-blind randomized controlled trial. J Rehabil Med 2018;50(2):200–8.

86. Evers S, Bryan AJ, Sanders TL, et al. The effectiveness of ultrasound-guided compared to blind steroid injections in the treatment of carpal tunnel syndrome. Arthritis Care Res (Hoboken) 2016. https://doi.org/10.1002/acr.23108.

87. Bang M, Kim JM, Kim HS. The usefulness of ultrasonography to diagnose the early stage of carpal tunnel syndrome in proximal to the carpal tunnel inlet: A prospective study. Medicine (Baltimore) 2019;98(26):e16039.

88. Ozsoy-Unubol T, Bahar-Ozdemir Y, Yagci I. Diagnosis and grading of carpal tunnel syndrome with quantitative ultrasound: Is it possible? J Clin Neurosci 2020;75(4):25–9.

89. Yin-Ting C, Miller Olson EK, Lee S-H, et al. Assessing diagnostic and severity grading accuracy of ultrasound measurements for carpal tunnel syndrome compared to electrodiagnostics. PM R 2020. https://doi.org/10.1002/pmrj.12533.

90. Manfield L, Thomas M, Lee SW. Flexor pollicis longus tenosynovitis in patients with carpal tunnel syndrome. Am J Phys Med Rehabil 2014;93(6):524–7.

91. Javed S, Woodruff M. Carpal tunnel syndrome secondary to an accessory flexor digitorum superficialis muscle belly: case report and review of the literature. Hand (N Y) 2014;9(4):554–5.

92. L'Heureux-Lebeau B, Odobescu A, Moser T, et al. Ulnar subluxation of the median nerve following carpal tunnel release: a case report. JPRAS 2012;65(4):e99–101.

93. Walter B, Ebert S, Sproedt J, et al. [Intraneural lipoma of the median nerve]. Handchir Mikrochir Plast Chir 2011;43(5):317–8.

94. Petrover D, Bellity J, Vigan M, et al. Ultrasound imaging of the thenar motor branch of the median nerve: a cadaveric study. Eur Radiol 2017;27(11):4883–8.

95. Altinkaya N, Leblebici B. Prevalence of persistent median artery in carpal tunnel syndrome: sonographic assessment. Surg Radiol Anat 2016; 38(4):511–5.

96. Bayrak IK, Bayrak AO, Kale M, et al. Bifid median nerve in patients with carpal tunnel syndrome. J Ultrasound Med 2008;27(8):1129–36.

97. Checa A, Hussain H. Sonographic assessment of a bifid median nerve and median artery in carpal tunnel syndrome. J Rheumatol 2011;38(8):1694–6.

98. Granata G, Caliandro P, Pazzaglia C, et al. Prevalence of bifid median nerve at wrist assessed through ultrasound. Neurol Sci 2011;32(4):615–8.

99. Salter M, Sinha NR, Szmigielski W. Thrombosed persistent median artery causing carpal tunnel syndrome associated with bifurcated median nerve: A case report. Pol J Radiol 2011;76(2):46–8.

100. Stavros K, Paik D, Motiwala R, et al. Median nerve penetration by a persistent median artery and vein mimicking carpal tunnel syndrome. Muscle Nerve 2016;53(3):485–7.

101. Stimpson JA, Gupta A. Persistent median artery (palmar type) and median nerve block in the forearm: observational study of prevalence. Reg Anesth Pain Med 2012;37(5):558–60.

102. Srivastava A, Sharma P, Pillay S. Persistent median artery thrombosis: A rare cause of carpal tunnel syndrome. Australas J Ultrasound Med 2015;18(2):82–5.

103. Fumière E, Dugardeyn C, Roquet ME, et al. US demonstration of a thrombosed persistent median artery in carpal tunnel syndrome. JBR-BTR 2002;85(1):1–3.

104. Jeon SY, Lee K, Yang W-J. Carpal tunnel syndrome caused by thrombosed persistent median artery - A case report. Anesth Pain Med (Seoul) 2020; 15(2):193–8.

105. Yalcin E, Onder B, Akyuz M. Trifid median nerve. J Hand Surg Eur 2011;36(9):812–3.

106. Shekhani HN, Hanna T, Johnson J-O. Lipofibromatous hamartoma of the median nerve: a case report. J Radiol Case Rep 2016;10(11):1–7.

107. Shapiro SA, Alkhamisi A, Pujalte GGA. Sonographic appearance of the median nerve following revision carpal tunnel surgery. J Clin Imaging Sci 2016;6(1):11.

108. Duetzmann S, Tas S, Seifert V, et al. Cross-sectional area of the median nerve before revision carpal tunnel release-A cross-sectional study. Oper Neurosurg (Hagerstown) 2018;14(1):20–5.

109. De Franco P, Erra C, Granata G, et al. Sonographic diagnosis of anatomical variations associated with carpal tunnel syndrome. J Clin Ultrasound 2014; 42(6):371–4.

110. Sun PO, Schyns MVP, Walbeehm ET. Palmaris longus interposition in revision surgery for recurrent and persistent carpal tunnel syndrome: a case series. J Plast Surg Hand Surg 2020;54(2):107–11.

111. Fong SW, Liu BWF, Sin CL, et al. A systematic review of the methodology of sonographic assessment of upper limb activities-associated carpal tunnel syndrome. J Chin Med Assoc 2020. https://doi.org/10.1097/JCMA.0000000000000415.

112. El-Karabaty H, Hetzel A, Galla TJ, et al. The effect of carpal tunnel release on median nerve flattening and nerve conduction. Electromyogr Clin Neurophysiol 2005;45(4):223–7.

113. Abicalaf CA, de Barros N, Sernik RA, et al. Ultrasound evaluation of patients with carpal tunnel syndrome before and after endoscopic release of the transverse carpal ligament. Clin Radiol 2007; 62(9):891–4.

114. Smidt MH, Visser LH. Carpal tunnel syndrome: clinical and sonographic follow-up after surgery. Muscle Nerve 2008;38(2):987–91.

115. Mondelli M, Filippou G, Aretini A, et al. Ultrasonography before after surgery in carpal tunnel syndrome and relationship with clinical and electrophysiological findings. A new outcome predictor? Scand J Rheumatol 2008;37(3):219–24.

116. Naranjo A, Ojeda S, Rúa-Figueroa I, et al. Limited value of ultrasound assessment in patients with poor outcome after carpal tunnel release surgery. Scand J Rheumatol 2010;39(5):409–12.

117. Tas S, Staub F, Dombert T, et al. Sonographic short-term follow-up after surgical decompression of the median nerve at the carpal tunnel: a single-center prospective observational study. Neurosurg Focus 2015;39(3):E6.

118. Kim JK, Koh Y-D, Kim JO, et al. Changes in Clinical symptoms, functions, and the median nerve cross-sectional area at the carpal tunnel inlet after open carpal tunnel release. Clin Orthop Surg 2016;8(3): 298–302.

119. Tajika T, Kuboi T, Endo F, et al. Relationship between morphological change of median nerve and clinical outcome before and after open carpal tunnel release: ultrasonographic 1-year follow-up after operation. Hand (N Y) July 2020. 1558944720937367.

120. Inui A, Nishimoto H, Mifune Y, et al. Ultrasound measurement of median nerve cross-sectional area at the inlet and outlet of carpal tunnel after carpal tunnel release compared to electrodiagnostic findings. Arch Orthop Trauma Surg 2016;136(9):1325–30.

121. Steinkohl F, Gruber L, Gruber H, et al. Memory effect of the median nerve: can ultrasound reliably depict carpal tunnel release success? Rofo 2017; 189(1):57–62.

122. Nitto A, Baur E-M, Gruber H, et al. [Concerning the Wrist-to-Forearm-Ratio of the Median nerve ultrasound is not a suitable method for assessing the success of a carpal tunnel release]. Handchir Mikrochir Plast Chir 2018;50(1):14–8.

123. Vogelin E, Nüesch E, Jüni P, Reichenbach S, Eser P, Ziswiler H-R. Sonographic follow-up of patients with carpal tunnel syndrome undergoing surgical or nonsurgical treatment: prospective cohort study. J Hand Surg Am 2010;35(9):1401–9.

124. Soyupek F, Yesildag A, Kutluhan S, et al. Determining the effectiveness of various treatment modalities in carpal tunnel syndrome by ultrasonography and comparing ultrasonographic findings with other outcomes. Rheumatol Int 2012; 32(10):3229–34.

125. Glowacki KA, Breen CJ, Sachar K, Weiss AP. Electrodiagnostic testing and carpal tunnel release outcome. J Hand Surg Am 1996;21(1):117–21.

126. Tan TC, Yeo CJ, Smith EW. High definition ultrasound as diagnostic adjunct for incomplete carpal tunnel release. Hand Surg 2011;16(3):289–94.

127. Tulipan JE, Kachooei AR, Shearin J, Braun Y, Wang ML, Rivlin M. Ultrasound evaluation for incomplete carpal tunnel release. Hand (N Y) 2019;27(2). 1558944719832040.

128. Yoshii Y, Ishii T, Tung W-L. Ultrasound assessment of the effectiveness of carpal tunnel release on median nerve deformation. J Orthop Res 2015;33(5): 726–30.

129. Motomiya M, Funakoshi T, Ishizaka K, Nishida M, Matsui Y, Iwasaki N. Blood flow changes in subsynovial connective tissue on contrast-enhanced ultrasonography in patients with carpal tunnel syndrome before and after surgical decompression. J Ultrasound Med 2017;36(suppl 1): 167–1604.

130. Nanno M, Kodera N, Tomori Y, Hagiwara Y, Takai S. Median nerve movement in the carpal tunnel before and after carpal tunnel release using transverse ultrasound. J Orthop Surg (Hong Kong) 2017;25(3). 2309499017730422.

131. Schelle T, Schneider W. [Is high resolution ultrasound of the median nerve helpful before reintervention after failed carpal tunnel surgery?]. Handchir Mikrochir Plast Chir 2011;43(5):313–6.

132. Kapuścińska K, Urbanik A. Efficacy of high frequency ultrasound in postoperative evaluation of carpal tunnel syndrome treatment. J Ultrason 2016;16(64):16–24.

133. Karabay N, Toros T, Çetinkol E, Ada S. Correlations between ultrasonography findings and surgical findings in patients with refractory symptoms after primary surgical release for carpal tunnel syndrome. Acta Orthop Traumatol Turc 2015;49(2): 126–32.

134. Erel E, Dilley A, Turner S, Kumar P, Bhatti WA, Lees VC. Sonographic measurements of longitudinal median nerve sliding in patients following nerve repair. Muscle Nerve 2010;41(3):350–4.

Preoperative Evaluation of Thenar Muscles in Carpal Tunnel Syndrome by Ultrasonography

Issei Nagura, PhD, MD[a],*, Takako Kanatani, PhD, MD[b],
Yoshifumi Harada, PhD, MD[b], Fumiaki Takase, PhD, MD[b],
Atsuyuki Inui, PhD, MD[c], Yutaka Mifune, PhD, MD[c],
Ryosuke Kuroda, PhD, MD[c]

KEYWORDS

• Carpal tunnel syndrome • Thenar muscle • Ultrasonographic evaluation

KEY POINTS

• We evaluated the thenar muscles in carpal tunnel syndrome by ultrasnography.
• The significant correlations of thenar muscles and the visual grading scale was found.
• We detected the recovery of the thenar atrophy after surgery by ultrasnography.

INTRODUCTION

Carpal tunnel syndrome (CTS) was a common entrapment neuropathy in the upper extremity. The main symptoms were the sensory disturbance of median nerve and thenar muscle atrophy. The thenar atrophy and dysfunction of opponens pollicis (OPP) were often seen in the advanced cases,[1,2] which were common in elderly patients.[3,4]

The incidence of thenar muscle atrophy in CTS was reported between 5% and 43%.[5–7] However, evaluation of thenar muscle atrophy has limited or no value as a diagnostic tool in CTS.[8] Because thenar atrophy was found in long-standing or neglected cases in the aged and the evaluation is based on subjective criteria. Then, some authors did not include thenar atrophy in their studies as a diagnostic tool.[9,10]

Although visual thenar evaluation was still used in several studies, especially for the assessment of surgical outcome, and it is usually classified as mild, moderate, or severe.[11,12] To standardize the visual evaluation, the simplified classification system was used or the same physician performed.[1–3,5,7] However, a certain level of bias may occur and the evaluation is not enough sensitive for assessment of the recovery.

In recent years, because of improvements in resolution, the simplicity of ultrasonography has found it gaining importance in the evaluation of soft tissues of the hand. Ultrasound imaging with measurement of the cross-sectional area and Power Doppler signals in the median nerve is a valuable tool for the diagnosis of CTS.[13,14] In this study, the usefulness of ultrasonographic evaluation as an objective evaluation tool for the clinical severity of CTS was assessed.

MATERIALS AND METHODS

A total of 85 patients with CTS who had a carpal tunnel release procedure (24 men and 61 women)

[a] Department of Orthopedic Surgery, Ako City Hospital, 1090 Nakahiro, Ako 678-0232, Japan; [b] Department of Orthopaedic Surgery, Kobe Rosai Hospital, 4-1-23 Kagoike-dori, Chuo-ku, Kobe 651-0053, Japan; [c] Department of Orthopaedic Surgery, Kobe University Graduate School of Medicine, 7-5-1 Kusunoki-cho, Chuo-ku, Kobe 6500017, Japan
* Corresponding author.
E-mail address: inagura0522@gmail.com

Hand Clin 38 (2022) 55–58
https://doi.org/10.1016/j.hcl.2021.08.004
0749-0712/22/© 2021 Elsevier Inc. All rights reserved.

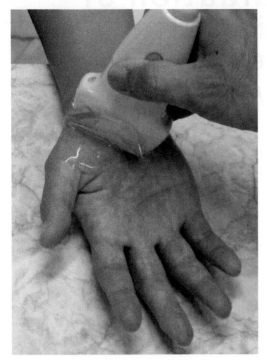

Fig. 1. At the time of measurement.

with a mean age of 67.4 years (range, 36–92 years) were included in this study. Ultrasonographic examination (SONIMAGE HS1 12 MHz, Konica Minolta INC, Tokyo, Japan) was performed to evaluate the abductor pollicis brevis (APB) and OPP muscles in a relaxed condition with forearm supination. To avoid pressure on the thenar muscle by the probe, it was covered with the gel pad (Sonocoupler, Toshiba, Tokyo, Japan) and then recorded with sufficient jelly (**Fig. 1**). The transducer was applied onto the palmar surface of the hand perpendicularly to the longitudinal axis of the first metacarpal bone. Both muscles were analyzed by measuring their thickness; the "APB depth" (from the inserted prominence of the OPP muscle above the first metacarpal bone to the palmar surface) and the "OPP depth" (from the ulnar prominence of the first metacarpal bone to the palmar surface of the OPP) (**Fig. 2**). Thenar atrophy was evaluated visually and classified by the visual grading scale[15]: none, mild, moderate, and severe. Also, distal motor latency (DML) was measured after stimulating the wrist, 7 cm proximal to APB. Antidromic sensory nerve conduction velocity (SCV) was measured at the wrist by stimulation at digit II. DML and SCV were analyzed to classify according to the electrophysiological severity scale[13]: stage I, normal DML and SCV; stage II, DML ≧ 4.5 ms and normal SCV; stage III, DML ≧ 4.5 ms and SCV less than 40.0 ms; stage

IV, DML ≧ 4.5 ms and nonmeasurable SCV; and stage V, nonmeasurable DML and SCV. The correlation of "APB depth" and "OPP depth" with the visual grading scale was analyzed by the chi-squared test ($P<.05$). The correlation of "APB depth" and "OPP depth" with the electrophysiological severity scale was analyzed by the Turkey-Kramer HSD test ($P<.05$).

RESULTS

The visual classification of these hands resulted in the following: none, 8; mild, 11; moderate, 40; and severe, 26. Preoperative electrophysiological assessment were as follows: stage II, 2 men and 2 women; stage III, 4 men and 7 women; stage IV, 13 men and 27 women; and stage V, 5 men and 25 women. As the severity of the visual grading scale increased, the averages of the "APB depth" and "OPP depth" decreased (**Table 1**). The significant correlations of both thenar muscles and the visual grading scale were found (men—APB [$P = .0008$] and OPP [$P = .049$]; women—APB [$P<.001$] and OPP [$P = .0013$]). However, in parallel comparing the severity of the electrophysiological grading, "APB depth" and "OPP depth" did not correlate (**Table 2**).

DISCUSSION

The occurrence of thenar atrophy is common in advanced CTS and thenar muscle atrophy is usually presented in electrophysiological severe cases.[1,2] It is a clinically significant sign because of its high association with decreased thenar muscle strength. In previous reports, MRI,[16] visual thenar evaluation,[11,12] and static hand prints[17] were used to evaluate thenar muscle atrophy; however, these have some disadvantages, which are as follows: MRI is expensive as routine assessment, visual thenar evaluation is inevitable

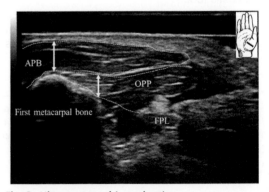

Fig. 2. Ultrasonographic evaluation.

Table 1
Correlations of thenar muscles and the visual grading scale

	Male APB (mm)	OPP (mm)	Female APB (mm)	OPP (mm)
None	12.5 ± 1.8	5.6 ± 1.3	8.1 ± 2.5	3.5 ± 0.4
Mild	8.2 ± 2.8	4.5 ± 1.2	8.1 ± 1.8	4.1 ± 0.9
Moderate	7.6 ± 2.1	4.5 ± 1.1	6.8 ± 1.9	3.7 ± 0.8
Severe	6.2 ± 3.5	3.9 ± 1.4	4.4 ± 1.3	3.1 ± 0.6

subjectivity, and static handprints are unable to evaluate the volume of muscle because of 2-dimensional evaluation. However, visual thenar evaluation was still used for the assessment of surgical outcome.[11,12] Most CTS patients are bilaterally affected and it is difficult to evaluate macroscopic atrophy compared with the contralateral side. Therefore, objective evaluation of the thenar muscle is essential.

Owing to the introduction of a high-frequency transducer, ultrasonography has been used for assessments of soft tissues and muscle conditions. Many physicians have reported its use for the measurement of muscle thickness and cross-section area of the median nerve.[13,14] Muscle movement and function can directly visualize in real-time. In addition, ultrasonographic evaluation costs lower compared with MRI and is easy to use regularly on outpatients. Grechenig and colleagues[18] reported the evaluation of all thenar compartments and their normal ultrasonographic appearance using ultrasonography. However, there were no articles focused specifically on the evaluation of thenar muscle atrophy using ultrasonography. Therefore, in this study, ultrasonography was applied in the quantification of thenar atrophy in CTS.

This article focused on the operated CTS cases and the thenar atrophy was found 90% in this study. As the severity of the visual grading scale increased, the average depths of the thenar muscle decreased. The significant correlations of both thenar muscles and the visual grading scale

were found. Therefore, thenar muscle atrophy could be evaluated using ultrasonography. The average depths of the thenar muscle were greater in men than in women. It is necessary to assess by gender in consideration of muscle volume. Female-OPP depths who did not show thenar atrophy were small because only 4 cases were evaluated.

However, the severity of the electrophysiological grading and both average depths did not correlate. Thenar muscle atrophy does not have a direct correlation with preoperative electrophysiological grading, although it is highly associated with severe CTS. The absence of thenar atrophy does not rule out CTS. The correlation of electrophysiological grading and clinical severity does not always reveal an exact match[8] and shows only a fair to moderate agreement for diagnosis.[16,19] So, what is the real incidence of thenar muscle atrophy and its clinical significance? Objective evaluation of thenar muscle atrophy using ultrasonography could solve this problem in the future.

This study has several limitations. First, the number of the patients was small because this study targeted only surgical cases, and need to use the normal cases as a control for accurate comparison. Second, this study did not evaluate about dominant versus nondominant hands, and need to be analyzed by increasing the number of the patients in the future. Third, this study did not evaluate the interobserver reliability and intraobserver reproducibility. Some authors reported

Table 2
Correlations of thenar muscles and the severity of the electrophysiological grading

Stage	Male APB (mm)	OPP (mm)	Female APB (mm)	OPP (mm)
II	13.0 ± 2.5	5.8 ± 1.5	4.5 ± 0	4.0 ± 0
III	9.0 ± 3.5	5.2 ± 1.1	7.5 ± 2.4	3.7 ± 1.0
IV	8.1 ± 2.3	4.5 ± 1.1	7.2 ± 2.0	3.7 ± 0.8
V	6.7 ± 2.6	3.8 ± 1.0	4.7 ± 1.6	3.2 ± 0.7

difficulty distinguishing a muscle using ultrasonography from surrounding muscles because of the change in echogenicity.[20]

This study demonstrated that the quantification of visual thenar muscle evaluation could be possible using the ultrasonographic evaluation. The ultrasonographic evaluation of thenar atrophy in CTS could be a useful tool for evaluating the thenar atrophy level. This technique is more precise than visual evaluation because it is a quantitative assessment. We believe that this technique can evaluate thenar muscles and follow muscle recovery over time.

CLINICS CARE POINTS

- Ultrasonographic assessment could be a useful to evaluate the thenar atrophy level in CTS.

REFERENCES

1. Gelberman RH, Pfeffer GB, Garbraith RT, et al. Results of treatment of severe carpal tunnel syndrome without internal neurolysis of the median nerve. J Bone Joint Surg Am 1987;69-A:896–903.

2. Norlan WBIII, Alkitis D, Grickel SZ, et al. Results of treatment of severe carpal tunnel syndrome. J Hand Surg Am 1992;17-A:1020–3.

3. Leit ME, Weiser RW, Tomanio MM. Patient reported outcome after carpal tunnel release for advanced disease: a prospective and longitudinal assessment in patients older than 70. J Hand Surg Am 2004;29-A:379–83.

4. Weber RA, Rude MJ. Clinical outcome of carpal tunnel release in patients 65 and older. J Hand Surg Am 2005;30-A:75–80.

5. Arons JA, Collins N, Arons MS. Results of treatment of carpal tunnel syndrome with associated hourglass deformity of the median nerve. J Hand Surg Am 1999;24-A:1192–5.

6. Edgell SE, McCabe SJ, Breidenbach WC, et al. Predicting the outcome of carpal tunnel release. J Hand Surg Am 2003;28-A:255–61.

7. Manktelow RT, Binhammer P, Tomat LR, et al. Carpal tunnel syndrome: cross-sectional and outcome study in Ontario workers. J Hand Surg Am 2004; 29-A:307–17.

8. D'Arcy CA, McGee S. The rational clinical examination: does this patient have carpal tunnel syndrome? JAMA 2000;283:3110–7.

9. Szabo RM, Slater RR, Farver TB, et al. The values of diagnostic testing in carpal tunnel syndrome. J Hand Surg Am 1999;24A:704–14.

10. Massy-Westropp N, Grimmer K, Bain G, et al. A systematic review of the clinical diagnostic tests for carpal tunnel syndrome. J Hand Surg Am 2000; 25-A:120–7.

11. Brown RA, Gelberman RH, Seiler JG, et al. Carpal tunnel release: a prospective randomized assessment of open and endscopic methods. J Bone Joint Surg Am 1993;75:1265–75.

12. Nagaoka M, Nagao S, Matsuzaki H. Endoscopic release for carpal tunnel syndrome accompanied by thenar muscle atrophy. Arthroscopy 2004;20: 848–50.

13. Lange J. Carpal tunnel syndrome diagnosed using ultrasound as a first-line exam by the surgeon. J Hand Surg Euro 2012;38:627–32.

14. Fowler JR, Maltenfort MG, Ilyas AM. Ultrasound as a first-line test in diagnosis of carpal tunnel syndrome: a cost-effectiveness analysis. Clin Orthop Relat Res 2013;471:932–7.

15. Kanatani T, Fujioka H, Kurosaka M, et al. Delayed electrophysiological recovery after carpal tunnel release for advanced carpal tunnel syndrome: a two-year follow-up study. J Clin Neuro 2013;30:95–7.

16. Britz GW, Haynor DR, Kuntz C, et al. Carpal tunnel syndrome: correlation of magnetic resonance imaging, clinical, electrodiagnostic, and intraoperative findings. Neurosurgery 1995;37:1097–103.

17. Tuncali D, Barutcu AY, Terzioglu A, et al. The thenar index: an objective assessment and classification of thenar atrophy based on static hand imprint and clinical implications. Plast Reconstr Surg 2006;117: 1916–26.

18. Grechenig W, Peicha G, Weiglein A, et al. Sonographic evaluation of the thenar compartment musculature. J Ultrasound Med 2000;19:733–41.

19. Atroshi I, Gummesson C, Johnsson R, et al. Prevalence of carpal tunnel syndrome in a general population. JAMA 1999;282:153–8.

20. Hodges PW, Pengel LHM, Herbert RD, et al. Measurement of muscle contraction with ultrasound imaging. Muscle Nerve 2003;27:682–92.

Sonography-Guided Peripheral Nerve Blocks for Hand Surgery

Amr Mohamed Aly, MD

KEYWORDS

- Distal nerve block • Ultrasound • Short procedures

KEY POINTS

- The proximal approaches to brachial plexus block are near to important structures, have late onset time and lead to loss of the motor control.
- Distal nerve blocks could be either done based on anatomical landmarks (with or without nerve stimulation guidance) or ultra-sound guided.
- Ultra-sound guided blocks are more efficient than anatomical landmark based for ulnar nerve blocks and less efficient for superficial radial nerve blocks in obese patients (BMI > 25 kg/m2).

INTRODUCTION

Trigger fingers, de Quervain tenosynovitis, and carpal tunnel constitute a large proportion of hand disorders. They usually are done as 1-day surgery that need short recovery duration equivalent to their short stay.

Regional anesthesia is superior to general anesthesia in short hand procedures for postoperative analgesia and reduced length of recovery and hospital stay besides being ideal for patients with chronic co-morbidities.[1]

The proximal approaches to brachial plexus block (supraclavicular plexus block, infraclavicular plexus block, and axillary block) are favored for most surgical procedures of the distal upper extremity, but their drawbacks include being anatomically near to important structures (phrenic nerve, pleura, and apex of the lung), late onset time, and loss of the motor control.[2] These drawbacks aroused the need for more distal nerve blocks, near the surgical incision and away from vital structures.[3]

Distal nerve blocks can be done based on either anatomic landmarks (with or without nerve stimulation guidance) or on ultrasound (US) guidance. This article describes upper limb distal nerve block techniques as part of a comparative study between anatomic landmark–based technique and US-guided technique in regard to block failure, time to sensory loss, vascular puncture, and nerve injury.

PATIENTS AND METHODS

Forty patients who were scheduled for outpatient trigger finger release, de Quervain tenosynovitis release, and carpal tunnel release at Ain Shams University Hospital (Cairo, Egypt) were included in the study, after informed consent. Exclusion criteria included age below 18 years, neurologic disease, and allergy to local anesthetics.

Patients were allocated randomly by computerized method into 2 groups: group 1, anatomic landmark–based nerve blocks (n = 20), and group 2, US-guided distal nerve blocks (n = 20). All the

Conflict of interest: The author declared no potential conflicts of interest with respect to the research, authorship, and/or publication of this article.
Funding: The author received no financial support for the research, authorship, and/or publication of this article.
Hand and Microsurgery Unit, Orthopaedic Department, Ain Shams University Hospital, 38 Abbasiya Square, Cairo, Egypt
E-mail address: dramrmoustafa@hotmail.com

Hand Clin 38 (2022) 59–64
https://doi.org/10.1016/j.hcl.2021.08.005

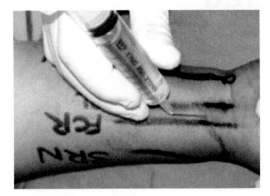

Fig. 1. Median nerve block.

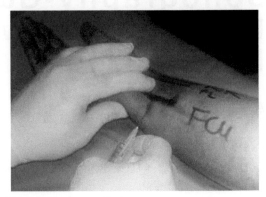

Fig. 3. Ulnar nerve block.

blocks were performed by the author, who was trained on musculoskeletal US.

Nerve blocks were performed in the induction area with no sedation. A mixture of equal parts 2% lignocaine and 0.5% bupivacaine buffered with (1:10) sodium bicarbonate was injected using a 10-mL syringe and 22-gauge (blue) needle. Each nerve was injected a volume of 5 mL.

The patient was placed in a supine position, with the arm 90° abducted and externally rotated. The skin was prepared with a disinfectant. In both techniques, aspirations were prior to injection to avoid intravascular injection, and any lancinating symptoms felt in the fingers prompted needle redirection.

GROUP 1: ANATOMIC LANDMARK–BASED NERVE BLOCKS

The skin was marked to outline the flexor carpi radialis (FCR), palmaris longus (PL), and flexor carpi ulnaris (FCU). The needle tip was bent to 45°. The insertion point for median nerve block was 2 fingerbreadths proximal to the wrist crease in the interval between the FCR and the PL tendons (**Fig. 1**). Aspiration was followed by smooth

injection of the local anesthetic, if any resistance redirection of the needle was performed. The needle then was redirected superficial to the FCR tendon, and injection of local anesthetic in the subcutaneous tissue was followed to block the palmar cutaneous branch (**Fig. 2**).

The insertion point for ulnar nerve block was 2 fingerbreadths proximal to the wrist crease just medial and deep to the FCU tendon (**Fig. 3**). The needle was advanced 5 mm to 10 mm. Aspiration was done, followed by local anesthetic injection. The needle then was inserted at the level of the ulnar styloid with the forearm in pronation position from dorsal to palmar till the FCU tendon, followed by local anesthetic injection to block the dorsal cutaneous branch of the ulnar nerve (**Fig. 4**).

The superficial radial nerve was blocked with the forearm in lateral position. The needle was inserted 3 cm proximal to the radial styloid in the subcutaneous plane (**Fig. 5**). The local anesthetic was injected during advancement of the needle from the lister tubercle dorsally till the radial artery anteriorly without piercing it.

GROUP 2: ULTRASOUND-GUIDED NERVE BLOCKS

With the forearm in supination position, a 10-MHz linear US probe (Sonosite, Bothell, Washington)

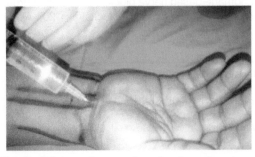

Fig. 2. .Palmar cutaneous branch of median nerve block.

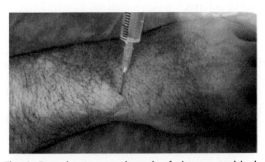

Fig. 4. Dorsal cutaneous branch of ulnar nerve block.

was placed perpendicular to the skin at the midforearm level (**Fig. 6**). The superficial radial nerve was identified just lateral to the radial artery. A 22-gauge needle was inserted in-plane from the radial side. Injection of the local anesthetic below and circumferentially around the nerve increased its contrast (**Fig. 7**).

The median nerve was inspected in the axial section with a honeycomb appearance, while the ulnar nerve was visualized at the same level just lateral to the ulnar artery. A 22-gauge needle was inserted in-plane from the radial side. As the needle tip was adjacent to the median nerve, aspiration was followed by injection of the local anesthetic, first below the nerve and then around the circumference (**Fig. 8**). The needle then was advanced just superficial to the median nerve toward the ulnar nerve. Aspiration was done followed by local anesthetic injection first below and then circumferentially around the nerve (**Fig. 9**).

MEASUREMENTS

Patient demographics and surgery type were recorded. Time to perform the block was measured when the needle penetrated the skin until the completion of the whole block. Time to sensory loss was assessed through pinprick testing at the dermatomal distribution of the blocked nerves at 1-minute intervals over the first 15 minutes. A successful nerve block was considered when no pain was felt by pinprick. Vascular puncture and nerve injury during and after block performance were recorded. Data were collected in a spreadsheet for the study.

ANALYSIS

The primary outcome measure of interest was complete nerve block at 15 minutes. A t test was used to compare continuous normally distributed data and Wilcoxon rank sum test was used for non-normally distributed data. Analysis was performed in GraphPad Prism 8.4.3 for Mac OS X (Graphpad Software, La Jolla, California). A 2-sided P value (<.05) was considered statistically significant.

RESULTS

Forty patients were enrolled in the study—19 were used for trigger finger release, 16 for carpal tunnel release, and 5 for de Quervain tenosynovitis release. Median, ulnar, and superficial radial nerves were blocked in all patients.

In group 1, the median age was 23 years (range 18–41 years); 15 were women and 5 were men. The average body mass index (BMI) was 22.4kg/m^2 (**Table 1**). There was failure of 40% (8 patients) of ulnar nerve blocks. Median and superficial radial nerves were blocked successfully in all cases (**Table 2**).

The median time to completion of the ulnar nerve block was 1.75 minutes per patient; the time to block onset was 7.5 minutes. The median

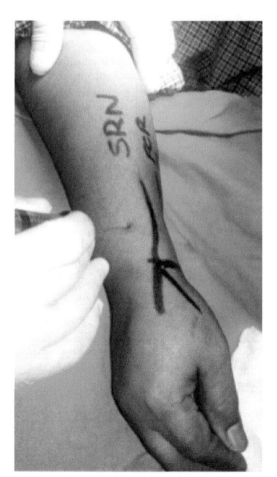

Fig. 5. Superficial radial nerve block.

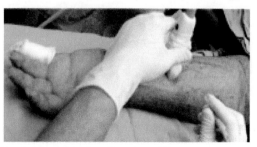

Fig. 6. US probe placed at the midforearm.

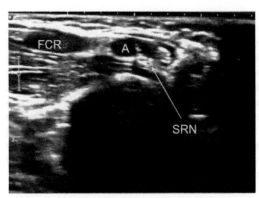

Fig. 7. US-guided superficial radial nerve block. A, radial artery; SRN, superficial radial nerve.

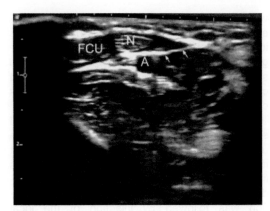

Fig. 9. US-guided ulnar nerve block. A, ulnar artery; N, ulnar nerve; Yellow arrows, needle.

time for a median nerve block performance was 2.5 minutes; the time to block onset was 5.2 minutes. The median time for a superficial radial nerve block performance was 1 minute; the time to block onset was 4.5 minutes. No complications were reported in the 20 blocked nerves.

In group 2, the median age was 31 years (range 20–45 years); 12 were women and 8 were men. The average BMI was 20.8kg/m². There was failure of 25% (5 patients) of superficial radial nerve blocks. Median and ulnar nerves were blocked successfully in all cases.

The median time to completion of the ulnar nerve block was 2.6 minutes per patient. The time to block onset was 6.8 minutes. The median time for a median nerve block performance was 2 minutes; the time to block onset was 12.2 minutes. The median time for a superficial radial nerve block performance was 5 minutes; the time

to block onset was 5.6 minutes. No complications were reported in the 20 blocked nerves.

DISCUSSION

The study demonstrated that time to perform nerve block was similar in both techniques except for superficial radial nerve, which was significantly shorter in the anatomic landmark–based technique (P value <.03). Both techniques had similar onset time for ulnar and superficial radial nerves, whereas median nerve block onset was significantly shorter in the anatowmic landmark–based technique (P value <.02).

Nerve block failure occurred in 40% of ulnar nerve blocks using the anatomic landmark–based technique, whereas US-guided nerve

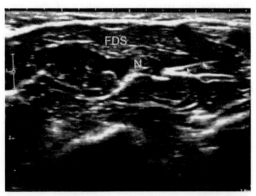

Fig. 8. US-guided median nerve block. FDS, flexor digitorum superficial; N, median nerve; Yellow arrows, needle.

Table 1
Patient demographics

	Anatomic Landmark–Based Nerve Blocks (n = 20)	Ultrasound-Guided Nerve Blocks (n = 20)
Sex (male:female)	5:15	8:12
Age (y)	18–41 (23)	20–45 (31)
BMI (kg/m2)	18–22 (20.8)	20–28 (26.4)
Surgery		
Trigger release	11	8
Carpal tunnel	6	10
de Quervain release	3	2

Values are mean (SD).

Table 2
Nerve block details

	Anatomic Landmark–Based Nerve Blocks (n = 20)	Ultrasound-Guided Nerve Blocks (n = 20)	P Value
Time to perform (min)			
Ulnar nerve	1.75 (1.5–2)	2.6 (1.4–3.2)	.3
Median nerve	2.5 (1.5–3.5)	2.0 (1.3–3.0)	.1
Superficial radial nerve	1.0 (0.75–1.5)	5 (3–7)	.03
Time to nerve block (min)			
Ulnar nerve	7.5 (4–9)	6.8 (5–10)	.1
Median nerve	5.2 (2–7)	12.2 (10–15)	.02
Superficial radial nerve	4.5 (2–8)	5.6 (3–7)	.07
Nerve block failure			
Ulnar nerve	8/20	0/20	.002
Median nerve	0/20	0/20	—
Superficial radial nerve	0/20	5/20	.02
Complications			
Ulnar nerve	0/20	0/20	—
Median nerve	0/20	0/20	—
Superficial radial nerve	0/20	0/20	—

Values are presented as medians and (range) or numbers.

blocks were not successful in 25% of superficial radial nerve blocks. Analysis of patient demographics showed that US-guided nerve block failures were performed in obese patients (BMI >25kg/m^2); this may explain the difficulty in viewing ultrasonographically the superficial radial nerve and failure of its block. Failure of ulnar nerve block using anatomic landmark–based technique is attributed to the blindness of the technique.

To the author's knowledge, this is the first randomized comparative study between anatomic landmark and US-guided distal nerve blocks. Sohoni and colleagues[4] performed a similar study but in 18 healthy volunteers. US-guided block was successful in 78% whereas anatomic landmark–based blocks were successful in only 56%. The investigators did not specify the success percentage of every nerve but stated the success of the whole block technique, which is considered a major limitation of their study.

A limitation of the study is that all nerve blocks were performed by a single consultant, who was not blind to the technique and results. This can be a source of bias in the results.

SUMMARY

Small hand procedures requiring median and superficial nerve blocks can be done using an anatomic landmark–based technique with a short time to perform and a short time for sensory block. Although US-guided blocks are more efficient for ulnar nerve blocks, this is attributed to the ability to visualize directly the spread of the local anesthetic in relation to the nerve.

CLINICS CARE POINTS

- Anatomical landmark based and ultrasound guided nerve blocks had similar onset time for ulnar and superficial radial nerves.

- Median nerve block onset was significantly shorter in the anatomical landmark-based technique.

- Ultrasound guided nerve blocks was not successful in 25% of superficial radial nerve blocks.

- Small hand procedures requiring median and superficial radial nerve blocks can be done using anatomical landmark-based technique with a short time to perform and short time for sensory block.

- U/S guided blocks are more efficient for ulnar nerve blocks.

REFERENCES

1. Neal JM, Gerancher JC, Hebl JR, et al. Upper extremity regional anesthesia. Reg Anesth Pain Med 2009;34(2):134–70.

2. Sehmbi H, Shah UJ, Madjdpour C, et al. Ultrasound guided distal peripheral nerve block of the upper limb: A technical review. J Anaesthesiol Clin Pharmacol 2015;31(3):296.

3. Liebmann O, Price D, Mills C, et al. Feasibility of Fore-arm Ultrasonography-Guided Nerve Blocks of the Radial, Ulnar, and Median Nerves for Hand Procedures in the Emergency Depart- ment. Ann Emerg Med 2006;48(5):558–62.

4. Sohoni A, Nagdev A, Takhar S, et al. Forearm ultrasound-guided nerve blocks vs land- mark-based wrist blocks for hand anesthesia in healthy volunteers. Am J Emerg Med 2016;34(4):730–4.

Cost-Effectiveness of Sonography-Guided Surgery

Ronny Kinanga, MD, Fabian Moungondo, MD, PhD*

KEYWORDS

- Percutaneous • Sonography • Surgery • Release • Cost-benefits • Carpal tunnel syndrome

KEY POINTS

- The surgical carpal tunnel procedure under sonography prevent intraoperative neurovascular injury.
- The sonography can also be used for carpal tunnel syndrome diagnosis and the surgical release.
- As a low-irradiation imaging technic, sonography can also be used for the trigger finger surgical procedure without skin incision.
- The percutaneous carpal tunnel procedure can be done without tourniquet and prevent from thromboembolism complication.

INTRODUCTION

Carpal tunnel syndrome (CTS) is the most frequent compressive neuropathy.[1] In Belgium, in 2018, there were 31,938 carpal tunnel releases (CTRs) performed with an annual direct reimbursement cost of 6,142,052 €. Most patients (64.4%) were women, and the median and average ages were 58 and 59.3 years, respectively. The vast majority of the operations (97.1%) were performed in an ambulatory day clinic.[2]

The classical surgical alternatives are Open and Endoscopic Carpal Tunnel Releases (OCTR and ECTR). In 2016, the American Academy of Orthopaedic Surgeons (AAOS) concluded that ECTR offers some benefits as compared to OCTR.[3] Sonography is now used more and more in CTS, for the diagnosis,[4] but also, by some physicians, during surgery. Already in 1997, Nakamichi suggested using sonography during CTR.[4] More recently, sonography has been proposed to guide the release of the transverse carpal ligament (TCL) using various endoscopic devices, or needles permitting sonography-guided percutaneous carpal tunnel release (PCTR). Several cadaveric studies have assessed the efficacy of PCTR.[5,6] Lecoq *and colleagues* reported in their series of 104 specimens, a total release of TCL in all cases. For 61 specimens, the complete release was obtained at first cutting movement.[6] In clinics, PCTR has been reported to be safe and could allow quicker return to daily activities and work.[7,8]

In 2017, PCTR has been introduced in our hospital. The operation is done in the operative room of the day clinic under local anesthesia. The first step of the procedure is a complete sonographic examination of the carpal tunnel region, to confirm the feasibility of the percutaneous sonography-guided release of TCL and to detect possible anatomic variations or abnormalities. Then, the upper extremity is prepared for an aseptic procedure and the release is performed using a bent catheter, under sonography guidance, with sterile gel and a sterile cover around the sonographic probe. At the end of the procedure, a metallic probe is used to confirm the completeness of the TCL release. The

Department of Orthopaedics and Traumatology, Erasme University Hospital, Université libre de Bruxelles, 808 Route de Lennik, 1070 Anderlecht, Brussels, Belgium
* Corresponding author.
E-mail address: Fabian.Moungondo@erasme.ulb.ac.be

Hand Clin 38 (2022) 65–73
https://doi.org/10.1016/j.hcl.2021.08.006

whole sonography-guided procedure takes about 10 minutes and then a compressive dressing is applied to prevent a postoperative hematoma. This dressing is removed on the first postoperative day and the patient can go back to his/her daily activities and resume light work. Note that during PCTR, no tourniquet is used, to allow good visualization of the vessels, particularly the ulnar artery and of the superficial volar carpal arch. Local anesthesia is also used because it is considered safer in this indication than general or regional anesthesia, the patient being able to describe a mechanical nerve stimulation during the procedure when the release motion is too close to it.

The aim of this study is to report the cost-effectiveness of PCTR as compared to OCTR and ECTR. The hypothesis was that PCTR was cheaper than OCTR or ECTR.

MATERIALS AND METHODS

This study is divided into 2 parts: an observational retrospective comparative study and a literature review. The research protocol has been approved by the Ethics Committee of the Erasme University Hospital (reference: P2019/571-CCB: B406201942256).

Part 1: Evaluation of Carpal Tunnel Surgery Direct Costs

All patients operated for CTS at our institution during the year 2019 were included in this study. One patient operated first by PCTR and later reoperated by OCTR in the same hand for persistent symptoms, 20 patients operated for CTS and concomitantly for another hand affection (ganglion, trigger finger, Dupuytren), and 4 patients with missing data were excluded in this study.

According to the preferences of patients and surgeons, 3 different techniques of surgery (OCTR, ECTR, and PCTR) were performed under 3 different techniques of anesthesia, general, regional (axillary or medio-ulnar block), and local. All PCTRs were performed under local anesthesia.

With the authorization of the billing department of our institution, all financial data related to these operations and anesthetics were recorded in an Excel file. All costs were expressed in Euro. The following parameters were collected: operating time duration (expressed in minutes), operating room occupation time (expressed in minutes), and direct costs related to the operation. These costs were categorized as:

- Costs of investment—corresponding to the hospital's investment for the acquisition of a tray of surgical instruments for OCTR and ECTR (including the endoscope for ECTR),

the purchase of the ultrasound machine for PCTR, and the acquisition of the arthroscopy column for ECTR.
- Disposable costs—these costs correspond to all disposable equipment used during the procedure (needles, surgical drapes, sutures, gloves, etc).
- Pharmacy costs—all drugs used during the procedure were counted, as well as the sling given to the patient to elevate the hand after the operation.
- Costs of occupation of the operating room— in the internal billing system of our hospital, this cost is fixed, regardless of the technique and the duration of the operation. The cost of occupation of the surgical room includes the cost of sterilization of the surgical instruments, estimated to be 50€ per set.

We did not consider in this study, neither surgeon fees, as in Belgium, these fees are the same whatever technique is used, nor the compensation expenses for the days off work after the operation, as we could not access these data.

Part 2: Literature Review

The literature review was carried out between January and May 2020 by consulting different databases: primary (JBJS, HC, AANA, JHS, HUES, and SMAR), secondary (PubMed, Cible +, ScienceDirect, and Google Scholar), tertiary (UpToDate, Cochrane Library, and INAMI), and quaternary literature (AAOS Guideline). The first part consisted of finding articles on CTS, the second part, in the selection of the articles. We used the PICO [Patient, Intervention, Compare and Outcome] method to establish the search equations to increase the chance of finding relevant articles. **Table 1** presents the equation research formulation. The combination of keywords (percutaneous, sonography, surgery, release, cost-benefits, and carpal tunnel syndrome) in the following Mesh term (((("Surgical Procedures, Operative" [Mesh]) AND "Carpal Tunnel Syndrome" [Mesh]) AND "Cost-Benefit Analysis" [Mesh]) AND "Sonography" [Mesh]) yielded no result. We modified the equation to another, which consisted in the determination of the cost-benefit of carpal tunnel surgery independently of the procedure. To not deviate from the objectives of our study and in view of the results obtained by the modified search equation, we also constituted several other search equations without MESH term by integrating the Boolean operators in several databases. All articles retained were selected according to the Strobe endpoint, for writing and reading observational studies.[9] With

Table 1
Equation of research using PICO model

Problem	Carpal tunnel syndrome
Intervention	Percutaneous carpal tunnel release sonography-guided
Comparative	Open carpal tunnel release
Outcome	Cost-effectiveness, economical cost

this different research equation, 2411 articles have been founded, and the following were excluded:

- All articles without 2 of the following keywords: percutaneous, sonography, surgery, release, cost-benefits, and carpal tunnel syndrome,
- All articles about cadaveric studies, anatomic studies, and studies comparing 2 nonsurgical techniques (like corticosteroid injections and orthosis),
- All articles dealing only with the endoscopic technique, regardless of the purpose of the study,
- All articles whose cost-effectiveness assessment was not included in the abstract or the results.

Of the 2411 articles, 13 articles were finally selected for the comparison of results and 5 others for the discussion.

RESULTS
Comparative Analysis of the Costs

A total of 141 patients (143 hands) were operated for CTS at Erasme University Hospital in 2019.

After exclusion criteria, 116 patients were included in the analysis: 35 men (mean age, 60 years) and 81 women (mean age, 54 years), 75 on the right side and 41 on the left side. Seventy-eight patients were operated by PCTR, 35 by OCTR, and 3 by ECTR. PCTR was performed by one single surgeon experimented in sonography (FM), OCTR and ECTR by multiple hand surgeons. Among the 116 operated patients, 29 were operated under regional anesthesia, 4 under general anesthesia, and 83 (including all PCTRs) under local anesthesia (**Table 2**). The average operative durations were similar for OCTR (15 ± 8 min) and PCTR (15 ± 6 min), inferior to those of ECTR (29 ± 10 min) (**Fig. 1**). The same difference was found for the total duration of occupation of the operating room (OCTR, 43 ± 17 min; PCTR, 47 ± 10 min; ECTR, 64 ± 34 min).

Investment costs
The investment costs were as follows: for PCTR, 42,129€ for purchasing the sonography device (42,000€), a needle holder (125€) and a buttoned stylus (4€); for OCTR, 1531.75€ corresponding to the purchase of a surgical hand surgery tray; and for ECTR, 68,052€ including the acquisition of an arthroscopy column (60,000€), the needed surgical instruments and endoscope (8052€).

Disposable costs
The common disposable to all CTS cases operated in our center, whatever surgical technique, included a surgical hand pack provided by Mölnlycke (Mölnlycke Healthcare, Göteborg, Sweden), which costed 35.37 €. For PCTR, the disposable cost was 6.23 € (cover for sonography probe 0.23 €, sterile ultrasound gel 3.5 €, 14G catheter 2 €, and Tuohy catheter 0.50 €); for ECTR, the

Table 2
Demographic data of patients grouped by anesthesia modality and surgical technique

Patients Recruited, N = 116			
Gender	Males: 35 (30.1%)		Females: 81 (69.9%)
Surgical technique	PCTR: 78	ECTR: 3	OCTR: 35
Side operated	Left: 41		Right: 75
Anesthesia modalities	General: 4	Regional: 29	Local: 83
Age	20–40 y: 15	41–60 y: 65	61–80 y: 26 81–90 y: 10

Distribution of Patients by Anesthesia Modalities and Surgical Technique, n = 116			
	PCTR	OCTR	ECTR
General anesthesia	—	4	—
Regional anesthesia	—	26	3
Local anesthesia	78	5	—

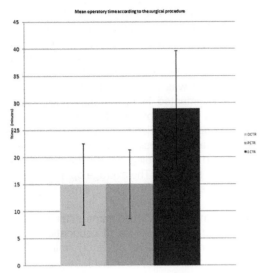

Fig. 1. Comparative operative durations.

cost of the disposable endoscopic knife was 201€.

Pharmacy costs

The costs of pharmaceutical drugs were on average 10.0 ± 2.9 € for PCTR, 23.2 ± 9.6 € for OCTR, and 19.0 ± 9.9 € for ECTR (**Fig. 2**). According to anesthesia modalities, the mean cost per patient was 10.55 ± 4.40 € under local anesthesia, 23.34 ± 8.79 € under regional anesthesia, and 29.36 ± 5.69 € under general anesthesia (**Fig. 3**).

Costs of occupation of the operative room

The costs for operative room occupation were the same in our institution, whatever surgical technique, despite the differences in room time occupation, 284.78€ per patient.

Instruments and disposable equipment used for percutaneous carpal tunnel release

Instruments and disposable equipment used in our hospital for performing PCTR are shown in **Fig. 4**. Two instruments (a needle holder and a buttoned probe), 3 needles, a 10 mL syringe, a probe cover, and sterile gel were needed to perform this surgery.

Literature Review

Postoperative functional improvement after percutaneous carpal tunnel release

In a study that included 194 patients, Logerlly and colleagues reported a mean postoperative functional and severity score of 13.8% in an OCTR group, compared to 14.2% in a minimally invasive group. The difference was not significant, both techniques were considered equivalent.[10] This score was established by a self-administered

questionnaire whereby patients recorded the severity of their symptoms and functional status. Each patient scored the functional status and severity of their symptoms in the preoperative consultation and then in subsequent postoperative consultations (up to 3 postoperative recordings were possible). These scores were then converted to percentages: 0 representing normal functioning or no symptoms, 100 representing severely restricted functioning or very severe symptoms.

Rojo-Manaute and colleagues reported a better Q-DASH score at 6 months postoperatively, in a study comparing PCTR to OCTR. The difference of grip strength was not significant, except the first week after the surgery where the force was better after PCTR. In the PCTR group, the patients recovered 5.3 times quicker full wrist flexion compared to the OCTR group.[11]

Nakamichi and colleagues used a satisfaction score to compare open and percutaneous techniques. Three weeks after surgery the PCTR patients were more satisfied than those operated by OCTR. Later, there was no difference in terms of satisfaction. These authors also reported that the sensitive discrimination measured by Semmens-Weinstein monofilament test was similar in both groups, and that the recovering of grip strength was not optimal in both groups.[7]

According to Petrover and colleagues in a non-randomized prospective trial comparing ECTR to OCTR, the Boston functional score improved significantly between 1 and 6 months in both groups.[12]

In 93 patients operated by PCTR, Chern and colleagues reported that the sensory disorder disappeared in 76.8% of patients 1 week postoperatively, and in 93.4% and 100% at 6 and 12 months, respectively, after the surgery.[13]

Effectiveness

In a study including 162 patients comparing OCTR to ECTR (one entrance portal), Saw and colleagues demonstrated a significant difference considering the return to work. In the ECTR group, the patients returned to work on average 8 days sooner (Confidence Interval (CI) 95%, 2-13 days). Considering the occupation time of the operating room, the tourniquet time and the time for the anesthesia, both techniques were similar. However, regarding the duration between skin incision and closure, ECTR was 2 minutes shorter than OCTR. In this study, there was no neurovascular lesion in either series.[14]

In 1997, Nakamichi and colleagues demonstrated in a prospective trial including 103 patients operated by PCTR or OCTR that there was no

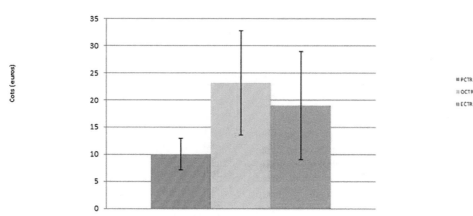

Fig. 2. Comparative pharmaceutical costs related to the surgery.

significant difference considering the sensitive discrimination and recovery of strength of abductor pollicis brevis muscle at 104 weeks after the surgery. However, in the PCTR group, there was significantly better grip and pinch strength after PCTR at 3, 6, and 13 weeks.[15]

In another nonrandomized study including 65 women operated either by PCTR or OCTR, Nakamichi *and colleagues* observed healing of the surgical wound on average after 1.4 days (IC 1–4 days) in the PCTR group, whereas it was on average 7.5 days (IC 6–10 days) in the OCTR group.[7]

Mc Shane *and colleagues* reported in a prospective study of 17 PCTR patients that the cross-sectional area of the median nerve diminished from 0.15 cm^2 preoperatively to 0.14 cm^2 in postoperative—the difference was statistically significant. In the same study, these authors found that the distal diameter of the median nerve increased significantly, from 0.14 cm to 0.21 cm postoperatively.[16]

In a prospective study on 129 patients operated by minimally invasive surgery using a groove probe, Benquet *and colleagues* reported that the mean duration of off work was 22.6 days and varied much from one patient to another (2–75 days). In the same study, these authors found that 90% of patients returned to work 3 weeks after the operation. The off-works duration was longer in

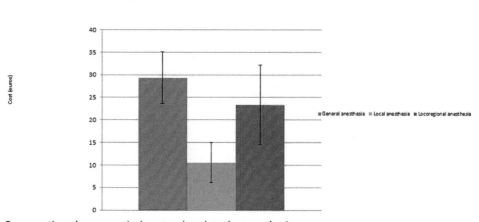

Fig. 3. Comparative pharmaceutical costs related to the anesthesia.

the hands worker group than in the nonhands worker group (23.2 ± 11.5 days vs 15 ± 7.8 days).[8]

Postoperative pain and complications

Nakamichi and colleagues[15] observed neither neurologic nor vascular complication after PCTR in their first study.

In a prospective randomized trial of 128 patients, Rojo-Manaute and colleagues observed that the mean duration of postoperative use of analgesics was shorter in the PCTR group than in the OCTR group. They also reported that the first- and third-week postoperative pains were 3 times less in the PCTR group than in the OCTR group.[11] Nakamichi and colleagues reported that postoperative pain was less in the PCTR group than in the OCTR group at 3 and 6 weeks. The postoperative sensitivity of the surgical wound was also less in the PCTR group at 3 weeks.[7] In the study of Chern and colleagues, there was moderate pain in 24.2% of patients 1 week after PCTR, the rate decreased to 6.6% after 2 months, and 1.1% after 12 months.[13]

Economic studies

Logerlly reported that the cost of CTS surgery varied between 65.23£ and 3971£, with an average of 800£ per patient. The mean cost of OCTR was 801.23£, the mean cost of minimally invasive surgery was 779.36£, the difference was not statistically significant.[10] Saw and colleagues compared the cost of ECTR and OCTR and reported higher costs with the first technique, 6482£ to purchase endoscopic devices and 82£ to purchase the single-use blade. However, according to the Confederation of British Industry, 1 day of off works costs on average 67£. Because ECTR had shorter return to work (8 days), the final gain for the society was 536£ per patient.[14]

Nakamichi and colleagues reported in their prospective study on 103 patients that the operative time duration was 54 minutes in the PCTR group and 48 min in the OCTR group. The mean cost of each surgery was 513$ in the PCTR group and 487$ in the OCTR group. The difference was mainly due to the particularity of the instruments used for PCTR surgery (26$ for the sonographic gel and the retractor).[15]

Rojo-Manaute and colleagues[11] used a blade hook, which costed 56.35 $ and can be reused several times.

Koehler and colleagues[17] reported that ECTR is 44% more expensive than OCTR (2759.70$ vs 1918.06$), and the difference is mainly related to the endoscopic blade. In the same study, they reported that the operative time was 44.8 minutes in the ECTR group and 40.5 minutes in the OCTR group.

DISCUSSION

Only one patient in the PCTR group had to be reoperated by OCTR for persistent symptoms, all others were markedly improved by the operation. Postoperative conversion of PCTR to OCTR is indeed quite low in all series. This high success rate is related to the excellent preoperative visualization of the anatomic structures offered by sonography.[4,18,19] Indeed, for the surgeon experienced in sonography, all structures are perfectly observed, including the location of the thenar branch and of the Berrettini medio-ulnar anastomosis, so sonographically guided surgery could be safer than open surgical dissection, especially by mini-open technique, and especially safer than endoscopy where only the TCL is seen from its deep surface. PCTR under sonography without tourniquet is in the opinion of the authors safer than ECTR and even safer than OCTR, provided that the surgeon master's sonography. The high success rate can also be attributed to the very minimally invasive technique that induces the least possible operative damage—only the TCL is sectioned, all other tissues are preserved.

Our hypothesis that PCTR is not only a safe and efficient method, but also cost-effective, has not been demonstrated, neither in our economic study nor in the literature review. However, it may still be cheaper, but only a prospective comparative trial including work compensation costs could demonstrate if it is the case.

The first source of costs is the investment needed to perform PCTR. PCTR compares unfavorably to OCTR, because of the cost of acquisition of the sonograph, but favorably to ECTR as the cost of the arthroscopy column and endoscope is higher. However, in some countries like Belgium, a medical fee code of sonography can be added to the medical fee code of the surgery and can allow reimbursing the investment. Another point to consider is that sonographs are already present in the operation rooms—to allow the anesthetists to perform sonography-guided nerve blocks, for example, so the equipment is frequently already available and financially amortized by other acts. Indeed, if in our study we had not considered the costs of acquisition of a sonography, considered in the study only for ECTR, but in fact used in our hospital for the 3 types of operations, PCTR for the surgeon and ECTR/OCTR for the anesthesiologists, then PCTR is the cheapest method. The same consideration applies to the arthroscopy column, used for wrist, shoulder, and knee arthroscopic procedures. It is also the case for the set of surgical instruments for hand surgery, used for other indications of hand surgery. For ECTR, a special fragile endoscope must be purchased, that cannot be used for other surgeries. This endoscope can break and then needs to be replaced. However, cheap portable sonographs are nowadays available on the market, but the authors insist that there should be no trade-off in the quality of sonographic imaging (high frequency) to allow perfect visualization of the hand tissues. If there is already a good sonograph in the operation ward, then the only investment necessary for PCTR is in our technique a buttoned stylus (see **Fig. 4**). Note that other surgeons use other instruments, for example, Petrover and Chern a sharped hook, Benquet a grooved director, and Markinson the Manos CTR system.[4,8,16,20,21]

The second source of costs, and one of the most important ones, is the duration of occupation of the surgical room. In our internal hospital billing system, these costs which include sterilization of the surgical instruments are the same, whatever the duration of CTS surgery (284.78€ per patient). A 2005 study of 100 US hospitals found that the costs of operating room occupation were on average $62/min (range, $22–$133/min), so a reduction of this duration, even by a few minutes, has a marked influence on the total costs of the operation.[22] The duration starts when the patient enters the room and ends when the patient leaves the room. We observed that the duration of occupation of the operative room was 43 min for OCTR, 47 min for PCTR, and 64 min for ECTR (the latter

evaluated in only 3 patients). Lecoq *and colleagues*[6] reported an operative time from 10 to 15 min in their cadaver PCTR study; Petrover *and colleagues,*[4] an operative mean time of 19 minutes and a mean time of occupation of the operating room of 38 min; Nakamichi *and colleagues,*[15] a mean operative time of 54 min in their PCTR group and 48 min in their OCTR group. So, the duration of occupation of the operative room seems to be similar in the published studies, and even slightly higher for PCTR than OCTR.

Can we reduce the duration of occupation of the operation room? In our study, the duration of the surgery itself was similar, 15 min on average, whether for PCTR or OCTR. These 15 min include in PCTR the local anesthesia. The nonoperative time is used, for PCTR, for the installation of the ambulant patient, for a preoperative nonsterile sonographic evaluation of the carpal tunnel region, and for accompanying the ambulant patient to the changing room, after completion of the dressing. In OCTR, the nonoperative time is used for the bringing of the regionally anesthetized nonambulant patient and installation in the operation room (at our institution, regional blocks are done in advance in a separate room), for the induction of general anesthesia, if this is the modality of anesthesia, then after the operation for wakening the patient and bringing him/her on a stretcher to the recovery room. For PCTR, the nonsterile part of the procedure could possibly be shortened, if sonography is only done under sterile conditions.

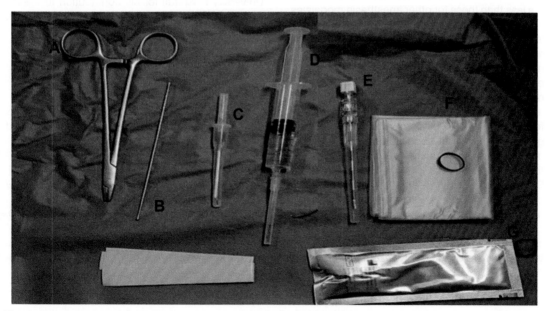

Fig. 4. Instruments used for PCTR in our center: (*A*) needle holder, (*B*) buttoned stylus, (*C*) 14G catheter, (*D*) syringe with anesthetic product, (*E*) Tuohy catheter, (*F*) cover for sonography probe, and (*G*) sterile ultrasound gel.

What would much change the operative costs would be to operate the patient in an outpatient clinic instead of in an operative room, which is perfectly possible given the fact that PCTR is done under pure local anesthesia with limited instrumentation, which is not possible for other techniques. We did not consider in this study another direct operative cost. PCTR can be performed by a single surgeon, without assistant, and even, if he/she opens sterile all material in advance, without a nurse. Obviously, OCTR and ECTR need at least a nurse in the operation room and if the anesthesia is not local, an anesthetist. Even though the OCTR can be done without an assistant, this is relatively unsafe and less efficient (longer operative time). In any case, PCTR, performed under local anesthesia, allows also to spare the costs of recovery room after regional or general anesthesia, frequently used for OCTR and ECTR—these costs were not considered in the present study.

The costs of the disposable and pharmaceutical products are in favor of PCTR, though the difference is modest with OCTR. We use two catheters (Tuohy and 14G). McShane *and colleagues* use an 18G needle,[4] Guo *and colleagues* use a metallic thread.[4] However, if for PCTR, a more sophisticated single-use instrument is used (eg, the Indiana Tome of Zimmer Biomet [cost: 225$]), then OCTR becomes cheaper. For Nakamichi *and colleagues*, PCTR surgery is more expensive because of the author using of many tools like sonographic gel and self-locking retractor.[15] We also observed that the pharmaceutical costs for local anesthesia are less than those for other anesthesia modalities.

The main source of reduction of costs of PCTR is probably for those patients still professionally active, the reduction of days off work. We could not study these indirect costs, and it is our experience in our academic hospital that most patients operated for CTS are not anymore working—active patients tend to choose private hospitals for CTS surgery. In this group of active patients, going back to work soon after the surgery can make a huge economical difference. However, there is no evidence yet in the literature that PCTR patients resume earlier their working occupations, but it can be assumed, as for ECTR, it has been demonstrated.

We recognize the limitations of our study. The size of our sample of patients was limited. The treatments were not randomized. Our protocol did not allow to measure the costs of recovery room nor the duration of days off work after the operation. Another limitation of the study is the low evidence level of the papers selected for the literature review. As there were few articles comparing PCTR to OCTR, we included also articles comparing ECTR to OCTR, and surgical technique to a nonsurgical technique.

SUMMARY

Our observational study does not show an economic advantage of PCTR. However, the lack of data on postoperative outcomes prevented us from determining a possible economic advantage in terms of earlier return of the patients to their professional activities, and we considered that a sonograph was needed only for PCTR, while actually a sonograph is also used for the anesthesiology in OCTR and ECTR. We anticipate also fewer iatrogenic complications after PCTR; neurovascular complications are reported after PCTR and ECTR and are costly. Further economic studies are needed, optimally through prospective randomized trials comparing functional results, complications, and costs between OCTR and PCTR.

We believe that PCTR will become quite popular in the coming years, as the morbidity is minimal, and the patient can resume his/her daily activities on the next day. The economic gains remain to be demonstrated.

AUTHOR CONTRIBUTIONS

R. Kinanga, F. Moungondo, and F. Schuind contributed to this article. The authors thank Frederic Schuind, MD, PhD (Past Head of the Department of Orthopaedics and Traumatology, Erasme University Hospital) for his contribution to the review of the paper and the acceptance of protocol.

CONFLICT-OF-INTEREST

The authors have nothing to disclose.

REFERENCES

1. Kothari MJ. Carpal tunnel syndrome: etiology and epidemiology. UpToDate; 2020.
2. Meeus P, Dalcq V, Beauport D. Variation des pratiques médicales: canal carpien. INAMI |Internet|. Available at: https://www.belgiqueenbonnesante.be/fr/variations-de-pratiques-medicales/systeme-nerveux/canal-carpien. Accessed December 20, 2019].
3. American Academy of Orthopaedic Surgeons. Management of carpal tunnel syndrome evidence-based clinical practice guideline. 2016. Available at: www.aaos.org/ctsguideline. Accessed May 7, 2020.
4. Petrover D, Richette P. Treatment of carpal tunnel syndrome: from ultrasonography to ultrasound

guided carpal tunnel release. Joint Bone Spine 2018;85:545–52.

5. Chern T, Wu K, Huang L, et al. A cadaveric and preliminary clinical study of ultrasonographically assisted percutaneous carpal tunnel release. Ultrasound Med Biol 2014;40(8):1819–26.

6. Lecoq B, Hanouz N, Vielpeau C, et al. Ultrasoundguided percutaneous surgery for carpal tunnel syndrome: a cadaveric study. Joint Bone Spine 2011; 78:516–8.

7. Nakamichi K, Tachibana S, Yamamoto S, et al. Percutaneous carpal tunnel release compared with mini-open release using ultrasonographic guidance for both techniques. J Hand Surg Am 2010;35(3): 437–45.

8. Benquet B, Fabre T, Durandeau A. Neurolyse du nerf médian au canal carpien par une voie mini-invasive. a propos d'une série prospective de 138 cas. Chir Main 2000;19:86–93.

9. Gedda M. French translation of the strobe Reporting Guidelines for writing and reading observational studies in epidemiology. Kinesither Rev 2015; 15(157):34–8.

10. Lorgelly P, Dias J, Bradley M, et al. Carpal tunnel syndrome, the search for a cost-effective surgical intervention: a randomised controlled trial. Ann R Coll Surg Engl 2005;87:36–40.

11. Rojo-Manaute JM, Capa-Grasa A, Chana-Rodriguez F, et al. Ultra–minimally invasive ultrasound-guided carpal tunnel release. J Ultrasound Med 2016;35(6):37–45.

12. Petrover D, Silvera J, De Baere T, et al. Percutanoeus ultrasound-guided carpal tunnel release: study upon clinical efficacy and safety. Cardiovasc Intervent Radiol 2017;40:568–75.

13. Chern T, Kuo L, Shao C, et al. Ultrasonographically guided percutaneous carpal tunnel release: early clinical experiences and outcomes. Arthroscopy 2015;31(12):2400–10.

14. Saw N, Jones S, Shepstone L, et al. Early outcome and cost-effectiveness of endoscopic versus open carpal tunnel release: a randomized prospective trial. J Hand Surg 2003;28(5):444–9.

15. Nakamichi K, Tachibana S. Ultrasonographically assisted carpal tunnel release. J Hand Surg 1997; 22(5):853–62.

16. McShane M, Slaff S, Gold J, et al. Sonographically guided percutaneous needle release of the carpal tunnel for treatment of carpal tunnel syndrome. J Ultrasound Med 2012;31:1341–9.

17. Koehler D, Balakrishnan R, Lawler E, et al. Endoscopic versus open carpal tunnel release: a detailed analysis using time-driven activity-based costing at an academic medical center. J Hand Surgery 2019;44(1):1–9.

18. Bianchi S, Demondion X, Bard H, et al. Ultrasound of the median nerve. Revue du rhumatisme 2007;74: 376–83.

19. Draghi F, Ferrozzi G, Bortolotto C, et al. Sonography before and after carpal tunnel release: video article. J Ultrasound 2020;23:363–4.

20. Guo D, Tang Y, Ji Y, et al. A non-scalpel technique for minimally invasive surgery: percutaneously looped thread transection of the transverse carpal ligament. Hand (N Y) 2015;10:40–8.

21. Markison R. Percutaneous ultrasound-guided MANOS carpal tunnel release technique. Hand (N Y) 2013;8:445–9.

22. Macario A. What does one minute of operating room time cost? J Clin Anesth 2010;22:233–6.

Sonography-Guided Carpal Tunnel Release

Isabelle David, MD

KEYWORDS

- Carpal tunnel syndrome • Interventional ultrasonography • Minimal invasive surgical procedures
- Ultrasound-guided surgery

KEY POINTS

- This is a new technique for carpal tunnel release thanks to recent improvement in the quality of ultrasound devices.
- The surgical technique is well described and consists in a wrist approach in a retrograde fashion under strict ultrasound control to transect completely the transverse carpal ligament.
- Outcomes of the first 150 patients, tips and tricks are presented and discussed.
- With a dedicated instrument, this is a safe and well-tolerated procedure, efficient, costless.

 Video content accompanies this article at http://www.hand.theclinics.com.

PREOPERATIVE CONSIDERATIONS

Carpal tunnel syndrome (CTS) is one of the most common neuropathies of the upper limb, and affects mainly manual workers. Its prevalence is approximately 5% of the population, and usually is diagnosed in the last active years (50–60 years old), with an increased incidence in women (4:1). Atroshi and colleagues[1] showed that the overall prevalence of neuropathy signs in the median nerve distribution is 14.4% (95% CI, 13.0%–15.8%).

They also determined that clinically certain CTS prevalence confirmed by electrodiagnostic tests (4.6% for women and 2.8% for men) was close to or somewhat lower than the true prevalence. CTS diagnosis is clinical, with typical symptoms including paresthesia, pain, and weakness in the median motor nerve distribution, often increasing in intensity at night. Ultrasound (US) and electromyography are used as means of additional evaluation and in poor clinically defined cases, if a differential diagnosis is needed. Once a diagnosis is confirmed, either medical or interventional treatment strategies can be used, the choice depending on the severity of the condition and the patient's decision. Among accepted severity criteria, authors find permanent amyotrophy of the thenar eminence due to its interrupted median nerve innervation, paralysis of thumb opposition, permanent paresthesia, and all forms of hyperalgesia.[2] For severe CTS patients (presence of clinical criteria, activity limitations, presentation of poor prognosis factors, and decreased quality of life) and for those who medical treatment failed, interventional options are preferred.[3,4]

SURGICAL TREATMENT OPTIONS

Surgery in CTS traditionally has been performed by an open approach carpal tunnel release (OCTR), but in the past 2 decades, many have opted by an endoscopic approach carpal tunnel release, owing to its reported advantages of reduced postoperative pain and rapid resumption of daily activities.[5–8] Nevertheless, the decision between endoscopic or open carpal tunnel release usually is based on surgeon and patient

Department of Hand Surgery, Belledonne Private Hospital, 83 Avenue Gabriel Péri, Saint-Martin d'Hères 38400
E-mail address: docteur.david@gmail.com

Hand Clin 38 (2022) 75–82
https://doi.org/10.1016/j.hcl.2021.08.007

preferences.[2] Another available option is the mini–open carpal tunnel release (miniOCTR), which emphasizes all minimally invasive advantages compared with OCTR and is superior concerning early postoperative pain.[9–11] These minimally invasive techniques present some disadvantages, including elevated cost of endoscopic equipment, the partially blind section of the retinaculum when carrying out miniOCTR, and the experience needed to operate the endoscope.

Over the past few years, the quest for an equally safe and effective alternative to OCTR has continued. Sonography long has been used for anatomic and severity assessments in patients with clinical CTS,[12–14] and the idea of CTS treatment under sonography guidance had its first clinical application in 2012,[15–17] although an attempt with its use already had been published in 1997. Sonography recently has been validated as a tool for accurate identification of vital anatomic structures and deemed safe for transverse ligament resection.[18] Efficacy of the transverse carpal ligament (TCL) section and percentage of postoperative complications have been shown to vary depending on the type of instrument used to carry out the procedure.[18–21]

After the development of a compact, easy-to-use scalpel for CTS surgical treatment, the author hypothesized that its use under US guidance would provide similar efficacy and tolerance compared with other CTS surgical treatment techniques. The main clinical outcome was the evaluation of grip strength 1 month after sonography-guided TCL release. The secondary endpoints included postoperative pain, persistence of nocturnal paresthesias, and resumption of daily work and driving activities as well as postoperative complications and subjective satisfaction.

AUTHOR EXPERIENCE

The present study was designed as a descriptive uncontrolled retrospective study (open label, single arm). This registry was carried out on 150 adult patients subjected to US-guided minimally invasive carpal tunnel release, completed with a new ligament transecting device. Participants' inclusion took place after clinical confirmation CTS. Inclusion criteria consisted of presence of a clinical syndrome (distal paresthesias in the median serve distribution areas, nocturnal numbness, weakness or atrophy of the thenar musculature, Tinel sign, positive Phalen test, and loss of 2-point sensory discrimination),[22] failure of medical management, and severe CTS at electromyography. Patients were excluded if another associated procedure was to be performed simultaneously or if the patient presented with additional upper limb pathology.

SURGICAL TECHNIQUE

All patients were operated on by the same orthopedic surgeon, specialized in hand surgery, and in similar operating room conditions. Once the patient was installed on the interventional table, with arm and forearm adequately positioned on a rest platform, the operator used a standard US probe (18 MHz) to adjust US parameters and mark the carpal tunnel limits (**Fig. 1**, Video 1). The first step concerned the setup, including the recommended cutaneous asepsis following by sterile drapes positioning. A tourniquet is useless. In this way, pulsing ulnar artery is easy to notice. Local anesthesia was carried out by the infiltration of 2-mL lidocaine, from 2 cm proximal of the wrist flexion line up to the distal limit of the volar transversal carpal ligament, completed by a regional ulnar and median nerve block at the forearm. The second step allowed the sonographic exploration in order to check all the different anatomic elements and variations. The third step focused on the section of the ligament and its control. The surgeon proceeded with a 3-mm to 5-mm transverse incision proximal to the wrist flexion crease, after the patient was completely insensible to local pain stimulus. Dissecting scissors were used to create an introduction path for a novel retrograde scalpel, specially designed for carpal tunnel release (Surgicut Ortho Release, reference ASOR12, Aspide Medical, La Talaudière, France) (**Fig. 2**). No trocar was required to gain access. At this point, US guidance was used to ensure that the mandrel protecting the scalpel was positioned correctly under the TCL inside the carpal tunnel, radially by the median nerve, and ulnarly by the hook of the hamate and ulnar vessels corresponding to the transverse safe zone. Once the device was in place, the protecting sheath was retracted and the scalpel was visualized. The surgeon placed it in horizontal position and progressed up to the hamate bone, which constituted the distal anatomic reference for ligament release. Finally, the cutting edge was placed vertically, and the TCL was transected completely in retrograde fashion, under strict US control. After the completion of this maneuver, the surgeon sheathed the scalpel and confirmed complete ligament section by US. Cutting steps were repeated if an incomplete section was observed. Once the device was removed, access incision was closed with a simple subcutaneous absorbable suture.

OUTCOMES

All parameters were registered during preoperative and at 1-month follow-up appointments. At

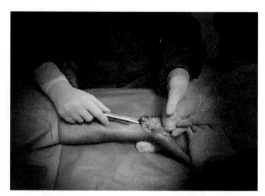

Fig. 1. External intraoperative image shows device placement.

inclusion, demographic data (age, gender, dominant hand, operated side, and degree of workload on professional activity) were obtained. Workload groups were built based on criteria accepted by the French High Authority for Health. Patients thus were placed in 1 of 4 groups: retired or currently unemployed (no workload), light workload (point load <10 kg, repeated load <5 kg), moderate workload (point load<25 kg, repeated load <10 kg), or heavy workload (point load >25 kg). To establish procedural efficiency, grip strength was analyzed before and at 1 month after surgery. Measurements were standardized by the use of a palmar dynamometer (Jamar Hydraulic Hand Dynamometer) and repeated 3 times per test in order to obtain an average of values, expressed in kilogram-force. Analysis reflected the percentage of postoperative grip strength recovery compared with preoperative values.

In parallel, data on postoperative pain were obtained on a standardized 1 to 10 visual analog scale. Time to nocturnal acroparesthesia resolution, and time to resumption of daily and work activities as well as driving also were registered. These were expressed as mean and SD values. Patients' subjective satisfaction regarding functional improvement was assessed on a scale of 1 (extremely unsatisfied) to 10 (extremely satisfied). Any procedure or suture related complications also were noted.

All parameters were analyzed using SPSS Statistical Package for the Social Sciences (IBM Corp. Released 2013. IBM SPSS Statistics for Mac, Version 25.0). Data were expressed as median and range of values, unless otherwise noted. Wilcoxon signed rank test was used for comparison between initial and final results of nonparametric variables, and Mann-Whitney U test or chi-square test was used for comparison of numerical or categorical data, respectively, between independent groups. Time to event was depicted graphically by means of a Kaplan-Meier (one minus survival) curve for resumption of daily activities, work, and driving. This retrospective study was approved by the ethics committee where patients were treated. After diagnosis, each patient was presented with different therapeutic options, and an informed consent form was voluntarily signed by those accepting the sonography-guided transverse ligament release.

RESULTS

Included in this study were 150 patients, aged between 23 years old and 88 years old (median: 59 years old). Data on gender, operated and dominant hand, and level of workload are expressed on **Table 1**. A significant majority were women ($P = .03$), and there were significant differences in terms of workload level per gender, with a strong correlation between the 2 (Spearman rho = 0.61). Of the 49 employed women, 38

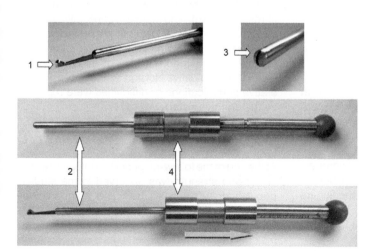

Fig. 2. External image shows the device and the cutting blade deployed (1, the blade; 2, the protecting sheath; 3, the slot of the sheath when the blade is inside; and 4, the central part of the device able to slide the blade out). Yellow arrow indicates the sliding direction of the device in order to go out the blade.

Table 1
Patient data

Studied criteria	Men	Women	All Patients (n = 150)
Gender, n (%)			
Men	—	—	55 (36.7)
Women	—	—	95 (63.3)
Age, median (range), y	60 (23–87)	58 (26–88)	59 (23–88)
Operated side, n (%)	*Dominant hand, n (%)*		
Right, n = 78 (52.0)			
Right	26 (47.3)[b]	46 (48.4)[b]	72 (48.0)
Left	2 (3.6)[b]	3 (3.2)[b]	5 (3.3)[b]
Ambidextrous	1 (1.8)[b]	—	1 (0.7)
Left, n = 72 (48.0)			
Right	24 (43.6)[b]	39 (41.1)[b]	63 (42.0)
Left	—	7 (7.4)[b]	7 (4.7)
Ambidextrous	2 (3.6%)[b]	—	2 (1.3)
Level of work charge, n (%)			
Light	5 (9.1)[b]	10 (10.5)[b]	15 (10.0)
Average	6 (10.9)[b]	38 (40.0)[b]	44 (29.3)
Heavy	15 (27.3)[b]	1 (1.1)[b]	16 (10.7)
Not applicable[a]	29 (52.7)[b]	46 (48.4)[b]	75 (50.0)

[a] Retried or without current professional activity.
[b] Percentage on similar gender population.

(77.5%) reported a moderate workload and only 1 (2%) a heavy workload, whereas of the 26 men still leading an active work life, 6 (23.1%]) stated a moderate workload and 15 (57.7%) had heavy workload functions (*P*<.01); 135 patients (90%) were right-handed but no differences were found between operated sides.

Median preoperative grip strength was estimated at 19.50 kgf (2–58). At 1 month postoperatively, subjects had recovered 73.7% (20%–650%) of the initial force, with a vast majority of participants exerting between 60% and more than 100% of their preoperative grip power (113 participants [75.3%]), as depicted in **Fig. 3**. A significant difference was found between preoperative and 1-month postoperative grip testing (*P*<.01).

Concerning immediate postoperative pain, 96.7% of subjects reported mild interference with functioning (visual analog scale 0–3), with more than 70% experiencing no pain. There were 4 patients with a visual analog scale of 4 (moderate pain),[23] 3.3% of the studied population.

Regarding the persistence of nocturnal acroparesthesias, only 1 patient (0.7%) reported persistent tingling of the distal extremities of the fingers after the first postoperative month.

Resumption of daily activities occurred for 90% of the patients at day 8. For 90% of the active population, work resumed 2 weeks after the procedure. Of the studied population, only 119 still were active drivers, and all were driving by the end of the first month of recovery (**Fig. 4**).

Among the patients, 71.9% were highly satisfied and 26.0% were satisfied with the postoperative final result. Three patients found that they were not entirely satisfied and attributed a score of 6 to the final result. No grade under 6 was attributed in this group of patients.

There were 3% reported complications on the first postoperative month, which included bilateral C6 cervicobrachial neuralgia (1 case), internal scar fibrosis (1 case), and hamate bone pilar pain (2 cases). Additionally, 7 patients presented with an inflammatory granuloma in reaction to suture material, 1 patient reported loss of sensibility, and another had sensitive incision scarring. No perioperative complications or difficulties were reported by the operating surgeon.

DISCUSSION

At the end of the follow-up period, significant recovery of grip strength was observed in the studied population. Additionally, pain and acroparesthesias resolved promptly after surgery, normal activities took less than 2 weeks to resume for a large majority of patients, and no serious complications were observed during the first postoperative

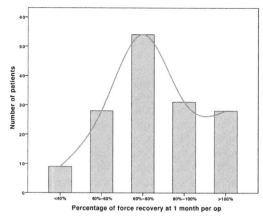

Fig. 3. Postoperative grip, 1 month. per op, per operative.

month. Procedural subjective satisfaction was high in approximately 98% of operated patients, indirectly reflecting good tolerance and functional results of US-guided release of TCL using a new compact scalpel.

Although grip strength and hand muscle atrophy are considered objective parameters reflecting functional status, there still are studies that do not measure and compare its preoperative and postoperative values. Besides, available reports often are contradictory regarding recovery of grip strength after transverse ligament release[16,24,25] When carrying out this study, it was judged unnecessary to use reference values for average grip strength[26] because they depend on numerous individual factors, such as subjects' age, current work activity and history, of manual efforts. Furthermore, because the study was retrospective, it lacked data to perform adequate comparison with published reference values, so it was decided to compare preoperative and postoperative values in order to determine functional outcome for this specific group of patients. The

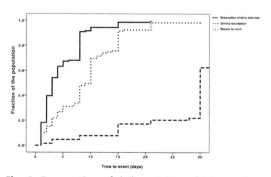

Fig. 4. Resumption of daily activities, driving and return to work postoperatively.

author observed a median recovery of ,greater than 60% of the preoperative grip strength for more than 75% of the patients at 1 month postoperatively, which reflects a significant improvement on functional status after percutaneous median nerve decompression. Moreover, the population showed excellent procedural efficacy regarding CTS acroparesthesia resolution, because only 1 of the patients experienced persistence of nocturnal tingling of the distal extremities of the fingers at the end of the follow-up period. The results are superior compared with the latest report by Petrover and colleagues,[27] who observed that 6 months after the surgery, 12% of their patients still presented with persistent paresthesia in the median nerve distribution. The use of US as an ancillary tool in CTS treatment allows for simultaneous visualization of TCL, median nerve, ulnar vessels, and the release instrument, which constitutes a clear advantage over endoscopic techniques.[18,20] In the study, a novel retrograde scalpel was used, specially designed for percutaneous carpal tunnel release, which allows for an incision reduction of up to 3 mm with simultaneous complete section of the TCL in all cases. Burnham and colleagues[18] and de la Fuente and colleagues[19] also performed minimal incision percutaneous releases with different tools and under US guidance. The first study was carried out on cadavers, impairing sonography vessel visualization and leading to overcautious section maneuvers, which increased the risk of incomplete release of the TCL with subsequent increase in CTS recurrence. Additionally, they used a threaded cutting loop with probable inferior stability compared with the author's scalpel. In the series, no remaining fibers were detected by US imaging on perioperative control after TCL section. No recurrences of CTS symptoms were observed during the follow-up period. de la Fuente and colleagues used a bulkier probe and a scalpel system that, although effective and without iatrogenic risks, required a larger skin incision with higher risk of scar pain and lower patient satisfaction, reducing advantages of a sonography-guided minimally invasive percutaneous approach.

Other surgical teams operating with a similar approach confirm that a retrograde section of the TCL through a proximal approach provides a safer and easier method of median nerve decompression, with excellent scar tolerance (less fibrous tissue and lower pressure compared to palmar incisions).[20,28] Observed tolerance and pain reduction probably led to an earlier return to work and a faster resumption of daily activities. Almost all patients in the study were observed carrying out normal daily activities on the first week after surgery and returning to work before the end of the second postoperative week. Rojo-Manaute and colleagues[29] reported a lower average for the resumption of daily activities, whereas Wang and colleagues[30] reported slightly superior delays on a study focusing on bilateral transverse ligament releases. Other investigators reported even longer sick leave periods.[31,32] This parameter is highly dependent on workload and surgeons' recommendations and difficult to compare between studies. In the author's practice, the author commonly advises a minimum leave of 2 days to 8 days, depending on expected workload, with reevaluation of period extension if needed. Patients usually are cautious after being subjected to TCL release, and some investigators even advise avoidance of any firm grip gesture before 6 weeks,[4] but in the author's case no such recommendations were made. Nevertheless, it was not until the end of the follow-up period that all the driving patients resumed the handling of steering wheels.

This has led to considering the importance of a more accurate evaluation of the reasons behind such a long delay as well as the need to determine what are the correct and advisable periods for resumption of activities after this procedure.

Failure of CTS surgical treatment is related not only to syndrome severity but also especially to delayed treatment leading to irreversible median nerve damage and even complex regional pain syndrome (CRPS).[4] In the author's study, all operated cases were diagnosed correctly and managed before irreversible nerve lesions appeared. Overall, excellent functional results are reported, associated with absence of pain in all patients at the end of the first postoperative month.

Bickel[33] published in a 2010 review, in which he concluded that patient satisfaction, and clinical as well as functional improvement after carpal tunnel surgery generally are quite high. Regarding subjective satisfaction, approximately 98% of the author's patients were satisfied with the procedure, similarly to other reports in the literature.[28] The few patients who were less satisfied presented with an inflammatory scar, which slightly decreased postoperative comfort. This was resolved in the months following the end of the study period.

Usual complications of carpal tunnel surgery include nervous, vascular, or tendinous damage; infections; and transient neurologic disturbances or CRPS. According to a recent state-of-the-art review on sonography-guided carpal tunnel surgical release, other investigators have seen complication rates decreasing significantly when using this technique, especially for what concerns postoperative infection and CRPS.[34] The author reported 3 patients with CTS-related complications in the first postoperative month and no perioperative difficulties nor complications.

Further investigation and longer follow-up period are necessary to determine the degree of implication of the US-guided procedure or the use of the novel TCL section instrument. The low percentage of postoperative complications, however, along with a surgical approach that allows for quick resumption of daily and work activities render the reported technique attractive in terms of overall patient benefit and costs. As suggested by other investigators,[34–36] authors currently are pursuing research to prospectively determine interventional times, postoperative complications, and functional outcomes in a new series of patients with a longer follow-up period and simultaneously establishing validation for its performance outside the operating room, further reducing treatment costs and increasing the technique's availability.

This is a retrospective study on cohort of 150 patients (level of evidence C). This report also is limited by the number of patients and by a short follow-up period. Concerning the latter, a longer follow-up could be of benefit to analysis, because further improvement over time is expected and later follow-up visits should show better functional status. With only 4 weeks of postoperative evaluation, CTS recurrences are impossible to determine. Another limitation resides in that all procedures were carried out but a single experienced operator limiting universal application of the technique. Results ideally should be confirmed by a randomized multicenter controlled trial evaluating safety and efficacy of percutaneous carpal tunnel release versus other standardized surgical approaches (open or endoscopic). Other parameters, such as hand muscle atrophy and recovery and relationship between section of TCL and recurrence of CTS, also would be useful to validate this technique further. US guidance constitutes a readily available, inexpensive, fast, and painless ancillary tool for carpal tunnel release, with the added advantages of intraoperative anatomic and lesion assessment. The author's results show that US-guided surgery for CTS using a novel retrograde scalpel is an efficient, well-tolerated procedure, which potentially will reduce treatment costs for CTS due to increased safety, by providing controlled median nerve releasing maneuvers, a faster recovery, and fewer complications. Randomized prospective studies on learning curve and procedural efficiency and tolerance on a larger patient series should be pursued in order to establish certainty of reported benefits.

Since this study, more than 1000 patients have been operated on by the same hand surgeon and the same procedure. Stiches now are useless and 3 adhesive tapes (Steri-Strips) are enough to close the wound avoiding an inflammatory granuloma. That is the only modification of this procedure.

CLINICS CARE POINTS

Pearls

- Explore with the probe the entire anatomic structures of the carpal tunnel before starting the procedure.
- Check the correct position of the device between the median nerve and the ulnar vasculonervous structures without flexor tendon interposition. Sometimes, the device has to be correctly reintroduced.
- Put the wrist in extension to place flexor tendon as deep as possible in the carpal tunnel.

Pitfalls

- If the antebrachial fascia is not open, the device will not be in a correct situation and not slide along the flexor tendon
- If the scalpel used for skin incision goes deeper, section of a superficial flexor tendon may occur.
- Without a second look after ligament section, a fibrous band may persist (including aponeurosis palm) and a constrictive localized stenosis on the median nerve realized.

DISCLOSURE

The author thanks Aspide Medical for lending freely the Surgicut device.

SUPPLEMENTARY DATA

Supplementary data related to this article can be found online at https://doi.org/10.1016/j.hcl.2021.08.007.

REFERENCES

1. Atroshi I, Gummesson C, Johnsson R, et al. Prevalence of carpal tunnel syndrome in a general population. JAMA 1999;282:153–8.

2. Scholten RJ, Mink van der Molen A, Uitdehaag BM, et al. Surgical treatment options for carpal tunnel syndrome. Cochrane Database Syst Rev 2007;(4): CD003905.

3. American academy of orthopaedic surgeons work group panel. Clinical guidelines on diagnosis of carpal tunnel syndrome 2007. Available at: www. aaos.org/research/guidelines/CTS_guideline.pdf.

4. Saint-Lary O, Rebois A, Mediouni Z, et al. Carpal tunnel syndrome: Primary care and occupational factors. Front Med (Lausanne) 2015;2:28.

5. Clapham P. Optimal management of carpal tunnel syndrome. Int J Gen Med 2010;3:255–61.

6. Oh WT, Kang HJ, Koh IH, et al. Morphologic change of nerve and symptom relief are similar after mini-incision and endoscopic carpal tunnel release: a randomized trial. BMC Musculoskelet Disord 2017; 18:65.

7. Ohno K, Hirofuji S, Fujino K, et al. Sonographic monitoring of endoscopic carpal tunnel release. J Clin Ultrasound 2016;44:597–9.

8. Vasiliadis HS, Xenakis TA, Mitsionis G, et al. Endoscopic versus open carpal tunnel release. Arthroscopy 2010;26:26–33.

9. Cellocco P, Rossi C, Bizzarri F, et al. Mini-open blind procedure versus limited open technique for carpal tunnel release: a 30-month follow-up study. J Hand Surg Am 2005;30:493–9.

10. Keith M, Masear V, Amadio P, et al. Treatment of carpal tunnel syndrome. J Am Acad Orthop Surg 2009; 17:397–405.

11. Wong K, Hung L, Ho P, et al. Carpal tunnel release. A prospective, randomised study of endoscopic versus limited-open methods. J Bone Joint Surg Br 2003;85:863–8.

12. Nakamichi K-i, Tachibana S. Distance between the median nerve and ulnar neurovascular bundle: clinical significance with ultrasonographically assisted carpal tunnel release. J Hand Surg 1998;23:870–4.

13. Wiesler ER, Chloros GD, Cartwright MS, et al. The use of diagnostic ultrasound in carpal tunnel syndrome. J Hand Surg Am 2006;31:726–32.

14. Wilder-Smith EP, Therimadasamy A, Ghasemi-Esfe AR, et al. Color and power doppler us for diagnosing carpal tunnel syndrome and determining its severity. Radiology 2012;262:1043–4. author reply 4.

15. Lecoq B, Hanouz N, Vielpeau C, et al. Ultrasound-guided percutaneous surgery for carpal tunnel syndrome: a cadaver study. Joint Bone Spine 2011;78: 516–8.

16. McShane JM, Slaff S, Gold JE, et al. Sonographically guided percutaneous needle release of the carpal tunnel for treatment of carpal tunnel syndrome. J Ultrasound Med 2012;31:1341–9.

17. Nakamichi K, Tachibana S. Ultrasonographically assisted carpal tunnel release. J Hand Surg Am 1997; 22:853–62.

18. Burnham R, Playfair L, Loh E, et al. Evaluation of the effectiveness and safety of ultrasound-guided percutaneous carpal tunnel release: a cadaveric study. Am J Phys Med Rehabil 2017;96:457–63.

19. de la Fuente J, Miguel-Perez MI, Balius R, et al. Minimally invasive ultrasound-guided carpal tunnel release: a cadaver study. J Clin Ultrasound 2013; 41:101–7.

20. Lecoq B, Hanouz N, Morello R, et al. Ultrasound-assisted surgical release of carpal tunnel syndrome: results of a pilot open-label uncontrolled trial conducted outside the operating theatre. Joint Bone Spine 2015;82:442–5.

21. Guo D, Guo D, Guo J, et al. A cadaveric study for the improvement of thread carpal tunnel release. J Hand Surg Am 2016;41(10):e351–7.

22. Graham B, Regehr G, Naglie G, et al. Development and validation of diagnostic criteria for carpal tunnel syndrome. J Hand Surg Am 2006;31:919–24.

23. Boonstra AM, Schiphorst Preuper HR, Balk GA, et al. Cut-off points for mild, moderate, and severe pain on the visual analogue scale for pain in patients with chronic musculoskeletal pain. Pain 2014;155: 2545–50.

24. Olsen KM, Knudson DV. Change in strength and dexterity after open carpal tunnel release. Int J Sports Med 2001;22:301–3.

25. Thurston A, Lam N. Results of open carpal tunnel release: a comprehensive, retrospective study of 188 hands. Aust N Z J Surg 1997;67:283–8.

26. Massy-Westropp N, Rankin W, Ahern M, et al. Measuring grip strength in normal adults: reference ranges and a comparison of electronic and hydraulic instruments. J Hand Surg Am 2004;29:514–9.

27. Petrover D, Silvera J, De Baere T, et al. Percutaneous ultrasound-guided carpal tunnel release: study upon clinical efficacy and safety. Cardiovasc Intervent Radiol 2017;40:568–75.

28. Rojo-Manaute JM, Capa-Grasa A, Rodríguez-Maruri GE, et al. Ultra-minimally invasive sonographically guided carpal tunnel release. J Ultrasound Med 2013;32:131–42.

29. Rojo-Manaute JM, Capa-Grasa A, Chana-Rodriguez F, et al. Ultra-minimally invasive ultrasound-guided carpal tunnel release: a randomized clinical trial. J Ultrasound Med 2016;35: 1149–57.

30. Wang AA, Hutchinson DT, Vanderhooft JE. Bilateral simultaneous open carpal tunnel release: a prospective study of postoperative activities of daily living and patient satisfaction. J Hand Surg Am 2003;28:845–8.

31. Hansen TB, Dalsgaard J, Meldgaard A, et al. A prospective study of prognostic factors for duration of sick leave after endoscopic carpal tunnel release. BMC Musculoskelet Disord 2009;10:144.

32. Ratzon N, Schejter-Margalit T, Froom P. Time to return to work and surgeons' recommendations after carpal tunnel release. Occup Med (Lond) 2006;56: 46–50.

33. Bickel KD. Carpal tunnel syndrome. J Hand Surg Am 2010;35:147–52.

34. Apard T, Candelier G. Surgical ultrasound-guided carpal tunnel release. Hand Surg Rehabil 2017;36: 333–7.

35. Henning PT, Yang L, Awan T, et al. Minimally invasive ultrasound guided carpal tunnel release: preliminary clinical results. J Ultrasound Med 2018;37(11): 2699–706.

36. Rajeswaran G, Healy JC, Lee JC. Percutaneous release procedures: trigger finger and carpal tunnel. Semin Musculoskelet Radiol 2016;20(5):432–40.

Safe Zones for Percutaneous Carpal Tunnel Release

Po-Ting Wu, MD, PhD[a,b,c,d], Tai-Chang Chern, MD[e], Tung-Tai Wu, MD, PhD[f],
Chung-Jung Shao, MD[g], Kuo-Chen Wu, MD[h], Li-Chieh Kuo, PhD[d,i],
I-Ming Jou, MD, PhD[j,k,*]

KEYWORDS

- Safe zone • Carpal tunnel release • Ultrasound • Percutaneous • Carpal tunnel syndrome

KEY POINTS

- Percutaneous carpal tunnel release is a trend that can be safely done under ultrasound guidance in strict accordance with the concepts of "safe zones."
- Using static bony landmarks, the transverse safe zone refers to the area between the median nerve and the hamate hook, and the longitudinal safe zone starts from 5 mm distal to the metacarpal metadiaphyseal junction to the 5 mm proximal to the midlunate within the transverse safe zone.
- Sometimes, anatomic variations such as the ulnar neurovascular bundle radial to the hamate hook and anomalous collateral vessels exist within the defined safe zones.
- Using the hydrodissection technique, the safety of the safe zones possible may be regained in cases with anatomic variations.

INTRODUCTION

Carpal tunnel syndrome (CTS) is one of the most common nerve entrapment syndromes.[1] Surgical carpal tunnel release (CTR) is recommended after failed conservative treatments. Open CTR is an effective technique using either a limited or a mini-incision.[2] The smaller incision has shown earlier functional recovery.[2,3] However, there is a concern that the procedure will be undergone blindly using a mini-approach. Endoscopic CTR (ECTR) provides clinical superiority to open CTR but invites a significant risk of nerve neuropraxia[4,5] that might be related to median nerve irritation or increased carpal tunnel pressure during blind insertion of the trocar.[5,6] In efforts to use real-time, continuous monitoring throughout the minimally invasive procedure, an ultrasound-guided CTR (UCTR) technique was developed. Different approaches and techniques proposed by several teams have reported clinically effective and safe outcomes.[3,7–19]

[a] Department of Orthopedics, College of Medicine, National Cheng Kung University, No. 1, University Road, Tainan 701, Taiwan; [b] Department of Orthopedics, National Cheng Kung University Hospital, College of Medicine, National Cheng Kung University, No.138, Sheng Li Road, Tainan 704, Taiwan; [c] Department of Biomedical Engineering, National Cheng Kung University, No. 1, University Road, Tainan 701, Taiwan; [d] Medical Device Innovation Center, National Cheng Kung University, No. 1, University Road, Tainan 701, Taiwan; [e] Tai-Chung Chern's Orthopedics Clinic, No.370, Bo Ai Road, Ping-Tong 900, Taiwan; [f] GEG Orthopedics Clinic, No. 253, Sec. 1, Dong Men Road, Tainan 701, Taiwan; [g] Department of Orthopedics, Tainan Municipal Hospital, No. 670, Chong De Road, Tainan 701, Taiwan; [h] Department of Orthopedics, Kuo's General Hospital, No.22, Sec. 2, Min Sheng Road, Tainan 700, Taiwan; [i] Department of Occupational Therapy, College of Medicine, National Cheng Kung University, No. 1, University Road, Tainan 701, Taiwan; [j] Department of Orthopedics, E-Da Hospital, No. 1, Yi Da Road, Kaohsiung 824, Taiwan; [k] School of Medicine, College of Medicine, I-Shou University, No.1, Sec. 1, Syue Cheng Road, Kaohsiung 840, Taiwan
* Corresponding author. Department of Orthopedics, E-Da Hospital, No. 1, Yi-Da Road, Kaohsiung 824, Taiwan.
E-mail address: ed109325@edah.org.tw

Hand Clin 38 (2022) 83–90
https://doi.org/10.1016/j.hcl.2021.08.008

Even though CTR is an effective procedure in open, endoscopic, or ultrasound-guided methods,[4,15] complications are present and potentially devasting. Most complications come from intraoperative technique errors,[20] especially in UCTR and ECTR approaches. UCTR requires substantial surgical experience and familiarity with the ultrasound-guided injection technique. Ultrasound provides real-time, dynamic monitoring,[21,22] but the view is still limited and interfered with by metal surgical instruments. Understanding the "safe zones" is essential to performing percutaneous CTR safely. This article provides a review of the anatomy of the safe zone and the UCTR techniques that can be used to prevent intraoperative complications.

SAFE ZONES IN ULTRASOUND-GUIDED CARPAL TUNNEL RELEASE
Related Anatomy

The carpal tunnel is defined by the carpal bone dorsally and the transverse carpal ligament (TCL) volarly. TCL is started proximally from the scaphoid to the pisiform and distally from the trapezium to the hamate hook.[23] The structures within the carpal tunnel are composed of both superficial and deep flexor tendons, the flexor pollicis longus tendon, and a median nerve that is the most volar structure (**Fig. 1**A, C). Around the carpal tunnel, the median nerve gives off 2 branches, the palmar cutaneous branch (sensory branch) and the thenar motor branch, which have the potential to be injured during CTR.[20] Although there are no major vessels except an anomalous median artery traveling with the median nerve within the carpal tunnel,[20] the ulnar artery and nerve run closely to the TCL and should be handled with caution during surgical release. Furthermore, the superficial palmar arch (SPA), a transverse anastomosis between the ulnar and superficial radial arteries, lies approximately 5 mm distal to the distal edge of the TCL[24] (**Fig. 1**B, D). One must be careful not to injure the SPA during distal release in an antegrade fashion or during palmar entry using a retrograde release.

Transverse Safe Zone

To avoid the violation of branches of the median nerve around the carpal tunnel, which usually arise from the radial side of the median nerve, the area between the median nerve and ulnar neurovascular structure is regarded as a "safe zone" for surgical release because there are no major neurovascular structures within this area (see **Fig. 1**A). This concept was first proposed by Nakamichi and colleagues in 1997 and has been

applied in ultrasound-assisted CTR for 50 hands in 50 patients without any complications.[7] However, the width of the safe zone proposed by Nakamichi and colleagues varied with the individual, where a safe zone that is too narrow ($\leq$3 mm) compromises the safety of surgical release.[25] However, we proposed the concept of a "transverse safe zone" using the static bony landmark, the hamate hook, instead of the ulnar neurovascular bundle, which is relatively mobile (see **Fig. 1**C). We defined the distance between the hamate hook and median nerve as the transverse safe zone. In a cadaver study, the width of the transverse safe zone was 5 mm on average (ranging from 4 to 8 mm), thus allowing insertion of surgical instruments and supporting the possibility of UCTR.[26] Currently, both the distances from ulnar artery and the hamate hook to median nerve, representing the working space for release instruments and the space for instrument insertion, respectively, should be preoperatively examined to evaluate the transverse safe zone. In most patients, the ulnar artery is ulnar to the hamate hook, but it is sometimes above or radial to the hook of the hamate,[20] which narrows the transverse safe zone. In our practice, the hydrodissection technique discussed later in this work is the preferred technique to perform UTCR safely in patients with a narrow transverse safe zone.

Longitudinal Safe Zone

During UCRT, an in-plane ultrasound monitor is recommended during the surgical release. In either an antegrade or a retrograde fashion, the longitudinal ultrasound imaging within the transverse safe zone is the major guidance during the entire procedure. In this imaging, there should be no major neurovascular structures above or beneath the TCL (see **Fig. 1**B, D). Therefore, the longitudinal safe zone makes it possible to prevent injury to the SPA, usually more than 5 mm distal to distal edge of the TCL and makes it possible to avoid incomplete release of the TCL. Even though the TCL can be comprehensively identified using recently developed high-frequency linear transducers (>13 MHz),[15] the introduction of a metal surgical instrument interferes with vision below the instrument. Furthermore, in the UCTR developmental period, a high-frequency transducer with a power of more than 13 MHz was not available.[7,11,25–27] In our previous cadaver study, static bony landmarks that can be easily identified using common high-frequency transducers correspond well to the actual location of the TCL and the SPA. Under longitudinal US imaging, the proximal edge of the TCL is very close to the midpoint of the

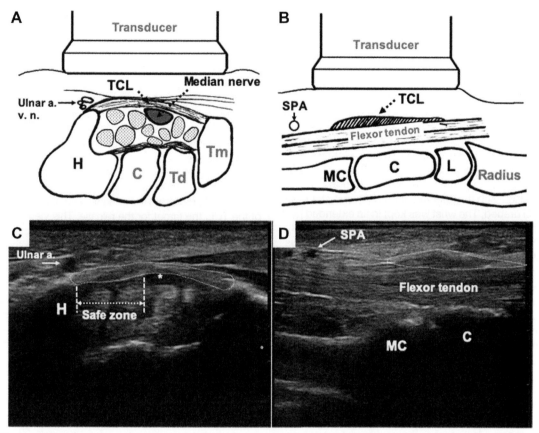

Fig. 1. Illustrations and ultrasound images of the transverse (A, C) and longitudinal (B, D) safe zones. The area circled by the broken line includes the TCL; *, the median nerve; a., artery; C, capitate; H, hamate; L, lunate; MC, metacarpal; n., nerve; Td, trapezoid; Tm, trapezium; SPA, superficial palmar artery; v., vein.

longitudinal axis of the lunate, and the distal edge of the TCL is very close to the metadiaphyseal junction of the metacarpal bone (see **Fig. 1**B). The differences between the bony landmarks under US imaging and the actual edge of the TCL are within 2 mm, which is virtually negligible in clinical practice.[26] The distance between the actual SPA to the actual distal edge of TCL is 11 mm (ranging from 6 to 16 mm),[26] following previous findings.[24] Therefore, we recommend that the CTR start from the metadiaphyseal junction of the metacarpal bone distally to the midpoint of the longitudinal axis of the lunate proximally[26] and should distally extend no further than 5 mm distal to the metacarpal metadiaphyseal junction.[11]

Other Considerations

Theoretically, surgical release can be performed safely after recognizing the transverse and longitudinal safe zones using ultrasound imaging. However, some anomalous anatomic variations exist in clinical practice. For example, there are sometimes visible collateral vessels above the TCL underneath the view of the longitudinal safe zone in patients receiving hemodialysis using the ipsilateral arteriovenous fistula. Previous traumatic or surgical insults may lead to similar anomalous collateral vessels. The hydrodissection technique can push the collateral vessels away from the defined longitudinal safe zone. If the safe zones cannot be guaranteed in either the transverse or the longitudinal view, we suggest that the UCTR should be converted to the open procedure. Another rare variation of the thenar motor branch of median nerve, type IC proposed by Lanz,[28] may challenge the concept of safe zones. However, up to the present time, there has been no such complication reported in the literature or in our practice using UCTR.

TECHNIQUES USED IN ULTRASOUND-GUIDED CARPAL TUNNEL RELEASE

Various UCTR techniques have been reported by several teams.[3,7–9,11–16,18,27] Here, we mainly describe our technique and briefly introduce other methods proposed by other teams. We usually perform UCTR in an operating theater for outpatients using only local anesthesia. We do not recommend the application of a tourniquet, which would mask the identification of safe zones.

Ultrasound Examination

In this example, high-frequency linear transducers were used (6–13 MHz; SonoSite, Bothell, WA, USA; or 4.2–13.0 MHz; GE Healthcare, Madison, WI, USA). The patient was prepared in the supine position with the affected hand and wrist sterilized and draped. The wrist was kept in an extended position at around 15° to 20° with padding (**Fig. 2**B). Other settings were the same as in our previous study.[11,12] After recognizing the median nerve, flexors tendons, TCL, ulnar artery, and targeted bony landmarks, including the hamate hook, the lunate, the third metacarpal, and the capitate, longitudinal imaging was initially conducted along the median nerve and centered at the capitate. Then, the transducer was moved parallel to the ulnar side

until the hamate hook was visible. The space between the median nerve and the hamate hook was the defined "transverse safe zone"[11,12,26] (see **Fig. 1**A, C). In this step, confirming if the ulnar artery or any pulsatile anomalous vessels are present in this area is crucial. If the transverse safe zone was determined to be "safe" (no ulnar artery, other pulsatile vessels, or visible nerve branches), the transducer was turned into the longitudinal view and held directly next to the hamate hook and centered on the capitate. In this view, the targeted bony landmarks, including the midportion of lunate and the metacarpal metadiaphyseal junction, were confirmed to represent the proximal and distal edges of the TCL, the target for the release. This view was the defined "longitudinal safe zone"[11,12,26] (see **Fig. 1**B, D). It was also necessary to ensure that the SPA was not within the longitudinal safe zone.

Entry

After confirming the safe zones, the UCTR was done using an in-plane wrist crease entry. We prefer the following instruments in this order: 21- and

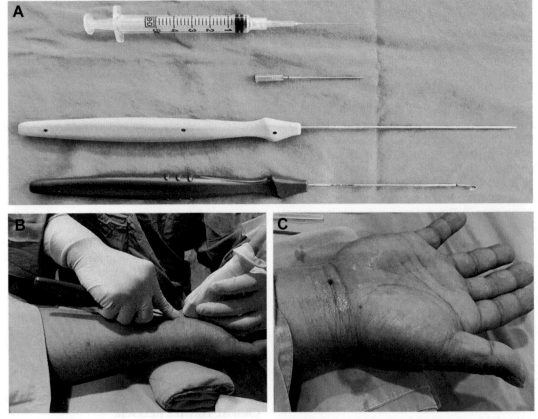

Fig. 2. Instruments used for ultrasound-guided carpal tunnel release in our practice: 5-mL syringe with 21-gauge needle, 18-gauge needle, and Ti-Chi hook knife set including a probe and a hook knife (*A*). Pictures taken during the clinical procedure (*B*) and postoperatively (*C*).

18-gauge needles, and Ti-Chi hook knife set (Aplus, Taipei, Taiwan) including a probe and a hook knife designed for UCTR (**Fig. 2**A, B). Palmar entry is another choice proposed by Nakamichi and colleagues[3,7] However, there are concerns related to the risk of damaging the SPA and sensitivity to a surgical scar on the palm as compared with one at the wrist crease.

Hydrodissection

The procedure began with infiltration using 1% lidocaine in a 5-mL syringe with a 21-gauge needle under the view of the longitudinal safe zone. With the exception of the entry, the infiltration, which usually requires 2 to 3 mL lidocaine, into the space between the TCL and the subcutaneous tissue is done from the entry to 5 mm distal to the metacarpal metadiaphyseal junction. When the local anesthetic fills and expands the targeted space, this is called hydrodissection (**Fig. 3**A, C). This procedure facilitated introducing the probe and the release instrument in the optimal position. When the ulnar artery or anomalous vessels were present within the transverse safe zone, this

technique also provided a safe route for UCTR using a certain amount of lidocaine (usually an additional 2–3 mL) to push the pulsatile vessel(s) away from this area. In such a clinical scenario, the effect of hydrodissection only lasts a few minutes, and the subsequent procedures must be completed within this period. This technique is demanding and requires substantial training.

Carpal Tunnel Release

After an 18-gauge needle was used to dilate the entry, the custom-made probe followed the track created by the hydrodissection. The probe plays 2 roles during a UCTR conducted in this manner: (1) it facilitates and confirms that the track is smooth for the later releasing instrument used in the safe zones (**Fig. 3**B, D) and (2) confirms the release is complete at the end of the procedure (**Fig. 4**B, D, E, F). After reconfirming that no pulsatile vessels or median nerves were present along the created tract (also within the 2 safe zones), the hook knife was then introduced along the track superficial to the TCL to distally reach the level of

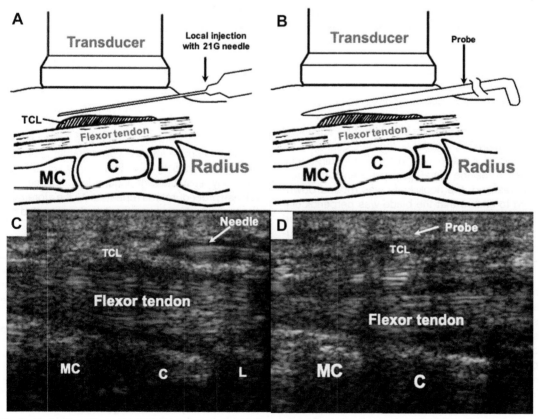

Fig. 3. Hydrodissection using 1% lidocaine was carried out along the space between the subcutaneous tissue and the TCL within the safe zones (*A, C*). The probe was introduced to confirm that the tract created by the hydrodissection was smooth for the hook knife following late (*B, D*). C, capitate; L, lunate; MC, metacarpal.

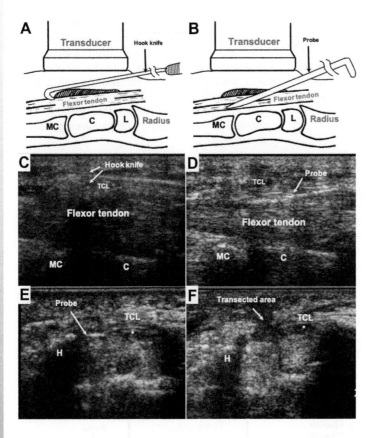

Fig. 4. The hook knife was advanced within the safe zones until it was 5 mm distal to the metacarpal metadiaphyseal junction, hooked onto the TCL, and withdrawn backward until it was 5 mm proximal to the midlunate (*A, C*). The probe was used to confirm adequate release, defined as unhindered movement of the probe from the subcutaneous space into the carpal tunnel (*B, D, E*). The transected area of the TCL was clearly visible in the transverse view (*F*). C, capitate; H, hamate; *, median nerve.

the metacarpal metadiaphyseal junction (**Fig. 4**A, C). In some cases, the junction between the distal edge of the TCL and the palmar fascia became thickened and required simultaneous release. However, the hook knife should not be advanced further than 5 mm distal to the metacarpal metadiaphyseal junction (within the longitudinal safe zone). Once the distal targeted area for release was reached, the hook knife was rotated downward to ensure that the blade was perpendicular to and hooked onto the TCL. CTR was carried out by pulling the knife retrogradely until the midlunate and extended proximally no further than 5 mm, if necessary.

Typically, the choices of the release instruments are subject to the surgeon's preferences and include hook knives with various designs,[3,10–12,16] the 18-gauge needle,[8] the scalpel blade,[14] the Gigli saw,[13] or specially-designed instruments, such as the basket punch,[7] the Kemis knife[15] and the Manos system.[9] When considering the SPA distal to the longitudinal safe zone and avoiding turning the knife around within the carpal tunnel, we prefer the retrograde release using a hook knife and the approach superficial to the TCL (outside the carpal tunnel).

Checking Release

The TCL is a very dense fibrous tissue that is remarkably resistant during probing and releasing. Therefore, adequate release was confirmed by the unhindered movement of the probe from the subcutaneous space into the carpal tunnel under the ultrasound imaging (see **Fig. 4**B, D, E). If there was any suspicion of incomplete release, the release procedure was repeated. All the aforementioned procedures were monitored and guided using real-time ultrasound observations.

Postoperative Care

After the operation, the entry wound (usually 1–2 mm) did not require suturing suture (**Fig. 2**C). It was covered with a dry dressing that could be removed the next day. Immobilization was unnecessary, and patients were encouraged to return to their normal life and work activity as tolerated.

CONTRAINDICATIONS

According to the literature, most authors excluded patients with previous surgeries on the affected hand in the clinical series. However, this does not mean a previous surgery should be a contraindication. Nakamichi and colleagues[7] proposed that once there is a hypertrophic flexor pollicis brevis or palmaris brevis extending into the safe zone in the ultrasound imaging, UCTR should not be performed. Kamel and colleagues[18] reported that when the distance from the median nerve to the ulnar artery is zero, or the distance between the distal edge of the TCL and the SPA is less than 2 mm, they exclude patients for UCTR. We agree that if there are visible neurovascular bundles in the previously defined transverse and longitudinal safe zones, UCTR cannot be performed safely. More specifically, we believe that the 2 zones are dynamic when using the hydrodissection technique. In idiopathic CTS, only an "unsafe" safe zone after hydrodissection is considered to be a contraindication for UCTR. In our early series, patients with recurrent CTS were excluded from UCRT.[11] With more experience, UCRT now is our first choice for idiopathic recurrent CTS due to advantages including minimal invasiveness and the fact that it is highly effective.

COMPLICATIONS

Even though anatomic variation exists, there have been no reports of neurovascular injury or wound complications during UCTR in the literature. In patients on hemodialysis who usually have anomalous collateral vessels in the upper extremities characterized by arteriovenous fistula, primary UCTR was done safely without any complications in 113 consecutive cases using our techniques.[17] In a 2-year follow-up of 641 hands in 376 patients, only 1 patient reported transient nerve palsy and recovered within 6 weeks.[19] Up to the present time, more than 4000 UCTR procedures have been performed by our team. There have been no permanent major neurovascular injuries reported in our records. However, we still emphasize that UCTR should not be done if the transverse and longitudinal safe zones cannot be guaranteed.

SUMMARY

In strict accordance with the concepts of safe zones, UCTR is an effective and reliable procedure for CTS. Substantial experience for ultrasound-guided injection and surgery is essential for safe UCTR.

CLINICS CARE POINTS

- As defined here, safe zone requires the route of release instruments to be away from vital structures including the median nerve and

its branches, the ulnar artery, the superficial palmar artery, and other collateral vessels. A preoperative ultrasound examination is essential.

- Using the hydrodissection technique, the safe zones become "dynamic" via pushing undesired vital structures away from the safe zones.

- If the transverse and longitudinal safe zones cannot be guaranteed, the ultrasound-guided carpal tunnel release should not be done.

DISCLOSURE

We thank the Taiwan National Science Council (grants: MOST 107-2314-B-006-065-MY3, MOST 110-2622-E-006-023, MOST 110-2314-B-006-022) and the National Cheng Kung University (grants: NCKUEDA 10903, NCKUEDA110006) for funding this work.

REFERENCES

1. Olney RK. Carpal tunnel syndrome: complex issues with a "simple" condition. Neurology 2001;56: 1431–2.
2. Cellocco P, Rossi C, Bizzarri F, et al. Mini-open blind procedure versus limited open technique for carpal tunnel release: a 30-month follow-up study. J Hand Surg Am 2005;30:493–9.
3. Nakamichi K, Tachibana S, Yamamoto S, et al. Percutaneous carpal tunnel release compared with mini-open release using ultrasonographic guidance for both techniques. J Hand Surg Am 2010;35: 437–45.
4. Sayegh ET, Strauch RJ. Open versus endoscopic carpal tunnel release: a meta-analysis of randomized controlled trials. Clin Orthop Relat Res 2015; 473:1120–32.
5. Shin EK. Endoscopic versus open carpal tunnel release. Curr Rev Musculoskelet Med 2019;12: 509–14.
6. Petrover D, Richette P. Treatment of carpal tunnel syndrome : from ultrasonography to ultrasound guided carpal tunnel release. Joint Bone Spine 2018;85:545–52.
7. Nakamichi K, Tachibana S. Ultrasonographically assisted carpal tunnel release. J Hand Surg Am 1997; 22:853–62.
8. McShane JM, Slaff S, Gold JE, et al. Sonographically guided percutaneous needle release of the carpal tunnel for treatment of carpal tunnel syndrome: preliminary report. J Ultrasound Med 2012;31:1341–9.

9. Markison RE. Percutaneous ultrasound-guided MANOS carpal tunnel release technique. Hand (N Y) 2013;8:445–9.

10. Capa-Grasa A, Rojo-Manaute JM, Rodriguez FC, et al. Ultra minimally invasive sonographically guided carpal tunnel release: an external pilot study. Orthop Traumatol Surg Res 2014;100:287–92.

11. Chern TC, Wu KC, Huang LW, et al. A cadaveric and preliminary clinical study of ultrasonographically assisted percutaneous carpal tunnel release. Ultrasound Med Biol 2014;40:1819–26.

12. Chern TC, Kuo LC, Shao CJ, et al. Ultrasonographically guided percutaneous carpal tunnel release: early clinical experiences and outcomes. Arthroscopy 2015;31:2400–10.

13. Guo D, Tang Y, Ji Y, et al. A non-scalpel technique for minimally invasive surgery: percutaneously looped thread transection of the transverse carpal ligament. Hand (N Y) 2015;10:40–8.

14. Lecoq B, Hanouz N, Morello R, et al. Ultrasound-assisted surgical release of carpal tunnel syndrome: results of a pilot open-label uncontrolled trial conducted outside the operating theatre. Joint Bone Spine 2015;82:442–5.

15. Apard T, Candelier G. Surgical ultrasound-guided carpal tunnel release. Hand Surg Rehabil 2017;36: 333–7.

16. Petrover D, Silvera J, De Baere T, et al. Percutaneous ultrasound-guided carpal tunnel release: study upon clinical efficacy and safety. Cardiovasc Intervent Radiol 2017;40:568–75.

17. Wang PH, Li CL, Shao CJ, et al. Ultrasound-guided percutaneous carpal tunnel release in patients on hemodialysis: early experiences and clinical outcomes. Ther Clin Risk Manag 2019;15:711–7.

18. Kamel SI, Freid B, Pomeranz C, et al. Minimally invasive ultrasound-guided carpal tunnel release improves long-term clinical outcomes in carpal tunnel syndrome. AJR Am J Roentgenol 2020;217(2): 460–8.

19. Wang PH, Wu PT, Jou IM. Ultrasound-guided percutaneous carpal tunnel release: 2-year follow-up of 641 hands. J Hand Surg Eur 2021;46:305–7.

20. Karl JW, Gancarczyk SM, Strauch RJ. Complications of carpal tunnel release. Orthop Clin North Am 2016; 47:425–33.

21. Wu PT, Lin CL, Tai TW, et al. Sonographically assisted percutaneous removal of screws in dynamization of the interlocking intramedullary nail. J Ultrasound Med 2013;32:319–24.

22. Wu PT, Lee JS, Wu KC, et al. Ultrasound-guided percutaneous radiofrequency lesioning when treating recalcitrant plantar fasciitis: clinical results. Ultraschall Med 2016;37:56–62.

23. Cobb TK, Dalley BK, Posteraro RH, et al. Anatomy of the flexor retinaculum. J Hand Surg Am 1993;18: 91–9.

24. Rotman MB, Donovan JP. Practical anatomy of the carpal tunnel. Hand Clin 2002;18:219–30.

25. Nakamichi K, Tachibana S. Distance between the median nerve and ulnar neurovascular bundle: clinical significance with ultrasonographically assisted carpal tunnel release. J Hand Surg Am 1998;23: 870–4.

26. Chern TC, Jou IM, Chen WC, et al. An ultrasonographic and anatomical study of carpal tunnel, with special emphasis on the safe zones in percutaneous release. J Hand Surg Eur 2009;34:66–71.

27. Rojo-Manaute JM, Capa-Grasa A, Rodriguez-Maruri GE, et al. Ultra-minimally invasive sonographically guided carpal tunnel release: anatomic study of a new technique. J Ultrasound Med 2013;32: 131–42.

28. Lanz U. Anatomical variations of the median nerve in the carpal tunnel. J Hand Surg Am 1977;2(1):44–53.

Percutaneous Sonographically Guided Release of Carpal Tunnel and Trigger Finger: Biomechanics, Clinical Results, Technical Developments

Fabian Moungondo, MD, PhD[a],*, Véronique Feipel, MD, PhD[b]

KEYWORDS

- Trigger finger • Carpal tunnel release • Sonography • Percutaneous release • Biomechanical study
- Cadaver study • Hand surgery

KEY POINTS

- Percutaneous sonographically guided procedures are increasing in hand surgery.
- Percutaneous release could potentially provide biomechanical advantage over open procedures in carpal tunnel and trigger finger release.
- No biomechanical studies have already compare the biomechanical effect of percutaneous carpal tunnel release with open technique.
- Optoelectronic motion capture system is reliable to assess tendon excursion in an in vitro model.
- A 3D kinematic model based on motion capture datas is propose to quantitatively compare percutaneous and open releases to treat carpal tunnel and trigger finger.

 Video content accompanies this article at http://www.hand.theclinics.com.

INTRODUCTION/HISTORY/DEFINITIONS/BACKGROUND

Improvement of sonography over the last 2 decades, with the superficial use of linear probes giving images of musculoskeletal superficial anatomic structures with high spatial and temporal resolution, now offers surgeons precise dynamic imaging of hand anatomy. Sonography is no longer reserved to radiologists, anesthesiologists, and rheumatologists; sonography is used by hand surgeons for diagnosis and progressively for interventional purposes like targeted injection, peroperative assessment,[1,2] and even percutaneous release.[3]

Trigger finger (TF) and carpal tunnel syndrome (CTS) are 2 common diseases that share the particularity of a simple basic principle in their surgical treatment: release of a ligament. A1 digit pulley and transverse carpal ligament (TCL) being relatively superficial anatomic structures, the use of sonography to guide their percutaneous release

The authors have nothing to disclose.

[a] Department of Orthopaedics and Traumatology, ULB Erasme University Hospital, Université Libre de Bruxelles, 808 Route de Lennik, Brussels 1070, Belgium; [b] Laboratory of Functional Anatomy, Faculty of Motor Sciences, Université Libre de Bruxelles, Campus Erasme CP 619, 808 Route de Lennik, Brussels 1070, Belgium
* Corresponding author.
E-mail address: fabian.moungondo@erasme.ulb.ac.be

Hand Clin 38 (2022) 91–100
https://doi.org/10.1016/j.hcl.2021.08.010
0749-0712/22/© 2021 Elsevier Inc. All rights reserved.

hand.theclinics.com

is one of the first surgical application of this technique in hand surgery.[3,4]

Percutaneous release of A1 pulley to treat TF is not a new technique. Blind percutaneous release was already described by Lorthior[5] in the middle of the previous century. However, blindly performed, percutaneous TF release carries a significant risk of neurovascular and/or tendon iatrogenic lesion, as well as a risk of incomplete A1 release or involuntary additional A2 opening. The use of sonography to guide this procedure seems to be of paramount help to prevent these complications.[6,7]

In the 1990s, Nakamichi and Tachibana[4] were the first to describe sonography to guide carpal tunnel release (CTR), and since then various more or less invasive surgical techniques have been presented.[8–12] Even if these procedures have some particularities in terms of skin incision size or location and in the feature of the instrumentation used to perform the release, they all share the same basic principle of releasing the TCL with as low as possible severance of the other soft tissues. The final goal is to perform a less invasive surgery that allows the patient to have a quicker recovery time with minimal complications and side effects. Clinical results of these kinds of procedures are very encouraging, and medical literature on this subject is growing fast.[3,4,6–12] However, the variability of the different techniques used and also the variability of the available study designs make it quite difficult to quantify the benefit of these new procedures, when compared with open release.

Minimally invasive release under sonography potentially allows the patient a quicker and better recovery of hand function, and this may be related to the duration of the operation (tourniquet time), to the size of the incision (small, or even no incision in percutaneous techniques), to the decrease of postoperative pain when the dissection is minimal, and also to the preservation of soft tissues other than the sectioned ligament, which would potentially decrease the phenomenon of bowstringing constantly observed after open release and leading to decreased strength.[13,14]

Clinical studies have demonstrated that carpal tunnel release is sometimes followed by a trigger digit onset. In a retrospective study of 140 CTRs, Hombal and Owen[15] described a TF onset prevalence of 21.9%. In contrast, in a retrospective study, Zhang and colleagues[16] observed that CTR release did not increase the overall risk of developing a TF, but the operation was modifying the distribution of the finger involved, the thumb being the finger most commonly affected after CTR instead of the middle finger, which was more often subject to TF before a CTR. The same distribution was observed by Goshtasby and colleagues[17] who found a TF prevalence of 6.3% after CTR in their retrospective study. These investigators observed that osteoarthritis and endoscopic procedure were independent risk factors to have a TF after CTR. Thumb carpometacarpal joint osteoarthritis was an explanation of predominantly observed thumb TF. Lee and colleagues[18] described a higher prevalence rate of TF after CTR, of 11.9% in a prospective study, wherein they also identified osteoarthritis as a significant risk factor for TF onset after CTR. Grandizio and colleagues[19] observed a prevalence of TF of 4% in nondiabetic patient 1 year after CTR. In their study the investigators found that the prevalence of TF after CTR was significantly greater in diabetic patient with 10% onset after 1 year. Another explanation of this TF onset and change of involved finger could be biomechanical. Flexor tendon bowstringing after CTR has been suggested as responsible for greater frictional force between flexor digitorum superficialis (FDS) tendon and the A1 pulley. The higher friction induced by the tendon bowstringing would then induce secondary changes and tenosynovitis.[15] This assertion was tested by Lee and colleagues[18] who observed a significant increase in volar FDS migration into the patient group with TF onset after CTR (2.5 ± 0.5 mm vs 1.8 ± 0.4 mm). These investigators suggested that because the cause of the TF is not the same after CTR, a higher failure rate of corticoid injection will be observed.[18] If this is the case, minimally invasive CTR under sonography, with possibly less flexor tendon bowstringing after the operation, could decrease the postoperative occurrence of TF.

There is therefore a necessity to assess the biomechanical consequences of techniques preserving the soft tissues other than the sectioned ligament, and possibly limiting bowstringing, when compared with open techniques. Bowstringing can be directly measured on postoperative MRI or sonographic images in patients, but given the anatomic variabilities and the precision of the measurements, sound conclusions cannot be anticipated from clinical studies. In the laboratory, it is easier to compare in the same specimen (for example during sequential release) fine biomechanical changes in flexor tendon moment arms. For the CTS, Kiristis and Kline[13] compared open and endoscopic techniques and observed that there was no significant difference between both techniques regarding flexor tendons excursion. To our knowledge there exists no biomechanical study comparing percutaneous and open release. For the TF, several biomechanical studies assessed the impact of A1 pulley release on the flexor tendon excursion. Hamman and colleagues[14] showed that the isolated A1 pulley release had minor effects with a drop to 96% on the flexor digitorum profundus excursion efficiency. The quantification of the tendon excursion combined with joint range of motion measurement allows to calculate the instantaneous tendon lever arms[20] and to define their modifications induced by the release. In the in vitro model of Lu and colleagues[21] tendon excursion was measured by the highly accurate linear variable differential transformer (LVDT), whereas the range of motion was recorded using an optoelectronic device. The investigators were able to calculate the changes of tendon moment arm during a continuous single finger motion, and to show that the release of the A1 pulley induced a statistically significant decrease of flexor tendon excursion efficiency (FDS and flexor digitorum profundus [FDP]) and an increase of flexor tendons moment arms with respect to the metacarpophalangeal joint (MCP).[21]

Another advantage of biomechanical studies conducted on anatomic specimens is to assess the new procedures for the possibility of iatrogenic lesions and to evaluate the completeness of the release.[22] The information obtained could then guide the choice toward the safest procedure.

The purpose of the present study is to present a biomechanical in vitro model that could be used to assess the biomechanical changes induced by carpal tunnel release and TF release. This model, once validated, could be useful to assess the efficiency of various new percutaneous techniques over open conventional CTR or TF procedures.

MATERIAL AND METHODS
Validation of Motion Excursion Measurement by Using the Vicon System

In preliminary study the comparison of the excursion measurement between LVDT (Solartron Inc, Oak Ridge, TN, USA) and Vicon system (Vicon Motion Systems, Oxford, UK) was performed. Two 20-mm-diameter reflective markers were fixed on a 2-mm-diameter polyamid cord. Each extremity of the cord was attached to a 500-g weight hanging freely from either side of 2 pulleys fixed on a frame. An LVDT was also fixed at one extremity of this frame in the axis of the 2 pulleys' line, and the polyamid cord was attached to its mobile part. The whole frame was put into the acquisition volume of 8 Vicon cameras, and a back-and-forth movement of the markers was manually

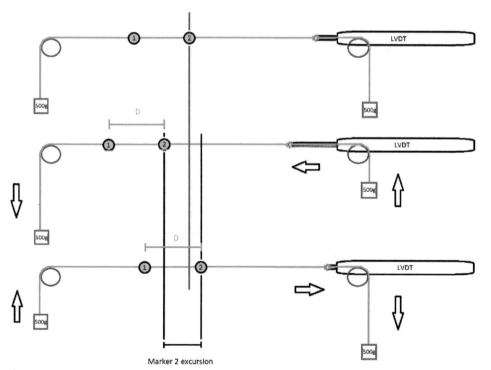

Fig. 1. Schematic representation of the setting used to compare the excursion values obtained from LVDT and Vicon system. Two reflective markers (*gray*) are attached on a polyamid cord (*green*). Two 500-g weights are attached on each extremity of the cord. Weights are suspended freely from 2 pulleys (*red*) attached on the frame. The cord is also attached on the mobile part of the LVDT. A back-and-forth excursion is induced by manually alternately pulling on each weight (*arrows*). Excursion values are obtained via LVDT and Vicon system, whereas the distance ("D") between the 2 markers is measured by using the Vicon system.

performed by pulling alternately on each weight. The movement was performed 10 times. The measurement of the marker excursion was performed simultaneously by using Vicon system and LVDT. The distance between the 2 reflective markers ("D") was also measured all along the back-and-forth movement by using the Vicon system (**Fig. 1**).

Biomechanical In Vitro Model

Fresh frozen cadaver hands were prepared in a standardized technique. A radiocarpal disarticulation was performed, preserving 10 cm of flexor and extensor tendons proximally to the wrist. Polyamid cords were sutured to all extensor and flexor (FDS, FDP, and flexor pollicis longus [FPL]) tendons of each finger by using Krakow strong sutures (Nylon 2-0) to allow a free load appliance (5 N).

Retrograde 1.5-mm K-wire pinning through distal interphalangeal (IP) and proximal IP joints in

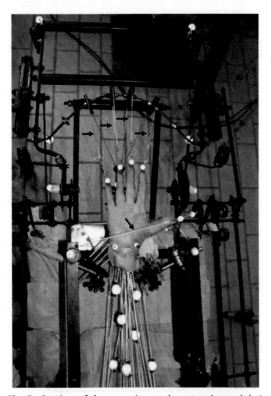

Fig. 2. Setting of the experimental anatomic model. A K-wire is introduced in a retrograde manner from the tip of the distal phalanx to the basis of the proximal phalanx to limit the motion to the MCP joint only. Two reflecting markers are fixed on each finger to quantify the MCP movement. A reflecting marker is also fixed on each tendon traction cord (*yellow cords*) to quantify tendon excursion. White cords (*arrows*) are attached from finger tips to the mobile part of the testing machine to induce passive finger movement.

long fingers and through the IP joint (for the thumb) was performed to allow only MCP joint movement.

Each specimen was mounted onto a motorized setup device by using external fixation pins screwed into the carpal bones, the palm plane being oriented with 30° of flexion relative to tendon's line of action (**Fig. 2**). The device allowed to put the fingers into cyclic passive MCP motion (0° to 90°) while loading fingers' flexor and extensor tendons with a free load of 5 N per tendon. Reflective markers were fixed on each tendon cord and on each finger (2 markers per finger) to allow motion capture into an acquisition volume defined by 8 infrared cameras of the Vicon optoelectronic system. The spatial coordinates of each reflective marker (attached to the tendons and finger) were recorded all along the finger's passive motions (**Figs. 3** and **4**).

Recording was performed for the following 6 states:

1. Intact
2. After percutaneous sonographically guided CTR
3. After open CTR (and visual control of the completeness of the percutaneous TCL release)
4. After wound closure
5. After percutaneous sonographically guided A1 pulley release
6. After open A1 pulley release (and visual control of the completeness of the percutaneous A1 pulley release).

Thumb motion was recorded separately in 2 configurations, with long finger fixed at 0° (DI 0°) and 45° (DI 45°) of MCP flexion.

After motion capture, reflective marker labeling was performed on Nexus software (Vicon Motion Systems, Oxford, UK), and a 3D kinematic model was built by using the LHP Fusion box software (http://lhpfusionbox.org, Brussels, Belgium).

Vectors were created from the moving reflective markers. Tendon marker motion allowed the quantification of tendon excursion by the measurement of vector modulus modification. Finger marker motion allowed the quantification of the finger MCP range of motion by defining the vector direction modification (**Fig. 5**, Video 1).

For each finger the following data were extracted from the virtual 3D kinematic model:

1. MCP range of motion (in degrees) as function of time.
2. Flexor tendon excursion (millimeters) defined as the distance between 2 positions of a single tendon reflective marker as function of time. Because the only moving joint was the MCP, this value reflected the bowstringing effect induced by the A1 pulley release.

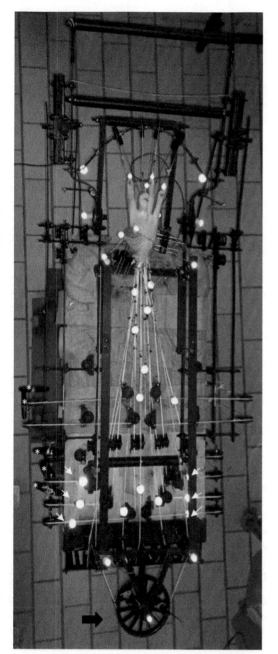

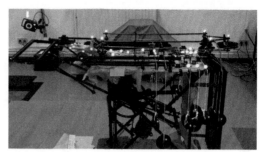

Fig. 4. Setting of the experimental anatomic model. Lateral view showing freely hanging weights (*asterisks*). Note one of the 8 motion capture system cameras at the upper left side of the picture (*arrow*).

3. Flexor tendon excursion area (mm) defined as the distance between a fixed point of the setup device (located at the level of the MCP joint of the corresponding finger) and the tendon reflective marker as function of time. Because the only moving joint was the MCP, this value reflected the bowstringing effect induced by the TCL release.

Statistical Analysis

Validation of motion excursion measurement by using the Vicon system

Excursion values obtained from LVDT and Vicon system were compared for the 10 back-and forth motions. Excursion lengths were subtracted to define the difference between both measurements. A correlation coefficient was calculated to compare the values obtained with both methods. The distance "D" was measured continuously by using the Vicon system to define the accuracy of the measurement of this segment during the movement.

Biomechanical in vitro model

Statistical analysis was performed on normalized tendon excursion data obtained by the division of the value of the measured tendon excursion by the maximal excursion obtained for the same digit. A 3-way repeated measures analysis of variance (ANOVA) with a Bonferroni posthoc test was performed for long fingers, considered factors being the arc of flexion of the MCP, the TCL state, and the A1 pulley state.

A 4-way ANOVA with a Bonferoni posthoc test was performed for the thumb. Considered factors were the fixed position of long fingers ($0°$ or $45°$), the arc of flexion of thumb MCP, the TCL state, and the A1 pulley state.

RESULTS
Validation of Motion Excursion Measurement by Using the Vicon System

The maximal difference between the excursion measured by the LVDT and the Vicon system

Fig. 3. Setting of the experimental anatomic model. Superior view showing the complex multiple pulley system that allows applying 5 N traction force on each digital flexor and extensor tendon via freely hanging weights (*asterisks*). Note that extensor tendon reflective markers are located at the rear left and right sides of the apparatus (*white arrows*). Long finger motion is induced by the motorized lever of the apparatus, whereas thumb movement is induced by the rotation of the wheel at the bottom of the picture (*black arrow*).

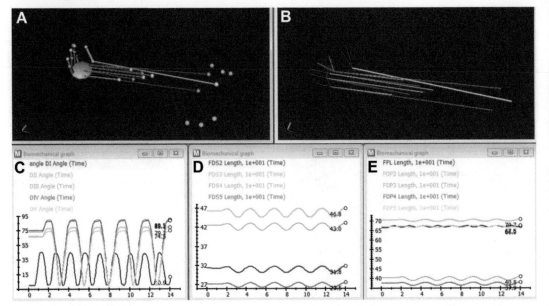

Fig. 5. Multiscreen display of the 3D kinematic model showing the complete simultaneous data recording. (*A*) 3D model of the hand built from reflective markers. (*B*) Vector building based on the 3D kinematic modeling. (*C*) Angle of MCP joint during the data acquisition period. (*D*) FDS excursion length (cm) induced by the finger movement. (*E*) FDS and FPL excursion length (cm) induced by the finger movement.

was 0.7 mm. The correlation coefficient between the excursion length for 10 measurements was 1.0 (**Table 1**).

The measurement of the distance ("D") between 2 markers obtained by using the Vicon system was stable all along the 10 movements with a standard deviation of 0.1 mm (**Table 2**).

Biomechanical In Vitro Model

A pilot study on 1 specimen was performed to assess the feasibility of this 3D kinematic model. Excursion of FDS and FDP tendon was measured all along the MCP flexion movement successively in the 6 different states. Flexor tendon excursion and flexion tendon area excursion were assessed.

On this single specimen the following observations were done. For what concerns the thumb, in the intact state, there was a decrease of FPL excursion when the long finger's MCP was extended from 45° to 0° (**Fig. 6**A). Interestingly, this effect of long finger flexion was not observed after CTR (**Fig. 6**B). The long finger flexor tendon excursion trend was finger specific, as well as the effect of CTR on tendon excursion. The fifth finger flexor tendon was the most sensitive to CTR. On this finger, there was a progressive increase of tendon excursion from percutaneous to open release with a light decrease of tendon excursion after wound closure. This effect was more marked on FDS (**Fig. 7**A) than FDP (**Fig. 7**B). Increased tendon excursion was

observed after percutaneous A1 pulley release and more after open A1 release (**Fig. 8**).

The area of tendon excursion was more modified by the CTR than after A1 pulley release. Changing of this parameter was also finger specific. The tendon excursion area was moving proximally after CTR. On the fifth finger, this migration was higher after open CTR than after percutaneous sonographically guided CTR, and skin closure was not restoring the percutaneous CTR area (**Fig. 9**). The change of tendon excursion after A1 pulley release seemed less marked.

DISCUSSION

A limitation of Lu and colleagues'[21] study design was that it allows the assessment of a single digit. The use of the very accurate LVDT to quantify tendon excursion has its own limitations because of the cumbersome setup of the device and because this measurement system does not allow cyclic back-and-forth motions easily. To overcome this difficulty we suggest instead the use of the optoelectronic motion capture system to assess not only fingers' motion but also the whole flexor's and extensor tendon's excursion by fixation of reflective markers on each of the tendons traction cords.

Although this adaptation would alleviate the setup device, the use of the optoelectronic system to quantify tendon excursion had to be compared with LVDT values before the validation of

Table 1
Mean of the excursion values obtained by linear variable differential transformer and Vicon system for 10 movements of reflective marker

Movement	Tendon Excursion (mm)		
	LVDT	Vicon	(Vicon)-(LVDT)
1	21.2	21.8	0.5
2	25.5	26.1	0.6
3	−49.0	−48.3	0.7
4	−35.9	−36.2	−0.3
5	−55.2	−55.9	−0.7
6	−26.8	−26.8	−0.1
7	15.9	16.4	0.5
8	−36.2	−36.7	−0.5
9	−56.1	−56.6	−0.5
10	−40.9	−40.6	0.3
Mean	−23.8	−23.7	0.1
SD	32.2	32.5	0.5
Correlation coefficient	1.0		

Because the displacement is performed manually, each excursion is different. The difference between the 2 measurement methods does not exceed 0.7 mm.

the proposed 3D kinematic model. The LVDT accuracy is 0.2 mm,[23] whereas the accuracy of the Vicon system depends on the size of the reflective markers, the speed of the motion analyzed, and the distance between the camera and the moving object. A system error of less than 2 mm is described, but the mean absolute error may decrease to 0.15 mm on static experiments in optimal configuration.[24] It seems essential to assess the accuracy of the measurements performed that are specific to the experimental condition of each laboratory.[25] The comparison performed between LVDT and Vicon system showed a good correlation for the excursion measurement with a maximal difference observed of 0.7 mm between the 2 techniques; this allows the use of Vicon system to assess tendon excursion when the expected modifications are more than 1 mm. The measurement of the distance between 2 reflective markers during the motion was also accurate by using the Vicon system with an SD of 0.1 mm for 10 movements. This finding allows the use of Vicon system to assess the modification of tendon excursion areas.

Another advantage of the presented experimental model is that the positioning of the specimen allows sequential releases without any modification of specimen setup that could be source of additional experimental errors. Then the modifications observed can reasonably be assumed to be the consequence of the surgical procedure performed.

Using this protocol, we conducted a pilot study on one specimen. No final conclusion can be drawn, but interestingly enough, we observed that the tendon excursion increased after CTR, but less after percutaneous than after open release. The same was observed after A1 pulley

Table 2
Mean of the distance "D" between 2 reflective markers during 10 movements

Movement	Distance "D" (mm)
1	115.6
2	115.6
3	115.7
4	115.7
5	115.8
6	115.7
7	115.7
8	115.7
9	115.7
10	115.8
Moy	115.7
SD	0.1

The measurement of this length was repeatable with an SD of 0.1 mm.

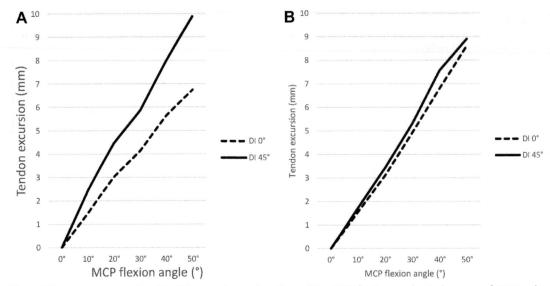

Fig. 6. Diagrams representing the FPL excursion as function of the MCP flexion angle. A decrease of FPL tendon excursion was observed when long finger MCP was at 0° of flexion (*dashed line*) (*A*). This decrease was not observed after CTR (*B*).

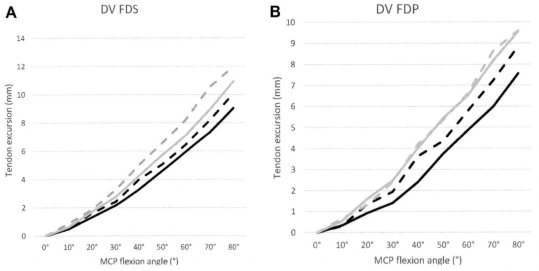

Fig. 7. Effect of CTR on the fifth finger FDS (*A*) and FDP (*B*) tendon excursion. Tendon excursion was progressively increasing from intact (*solid black line*) state to percutaneous release state (*dashed black line*) and from the latter to the open release state (*dashed gray line*). Skin closure (*solid gray line*) seemed to decrease the excursion at a level above that of percutaneous release state. This difference was more obvious on FDS than FDP tendon.

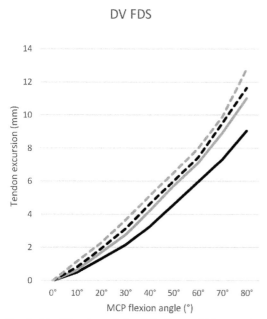

DV FDS

Fig. 8. Modification of the fifth finger FDS excursion with MCP flexion. Tendon excursion was increasing from the intact state (*solid black line*) to the sequential CTR (*solid gray line*), percutaneous A1 release (*black dashed line*), and open A1 pulley release (*gray dashed line*).

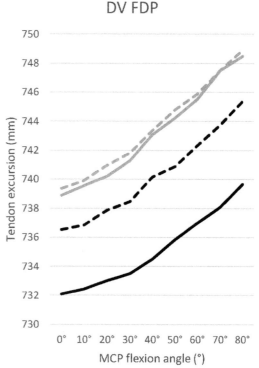

DV FDP

Fig. 9. Effect of CTR on FDP excursion of the fifth finger. The tendon excursion area was displaced proximally after percutaneous CTR (*dashed black line*) when compared with the intact state. Proximal migration of this excursion area was higher after open CTR (*dashed gray line*), and skin closure (*solid gray line*) does not restore the previous percutaneous CTR excursion area.

release. Another observation in this pilot study was the important modification of the tendon excursion area after CTR. We believe that our method is a good way to quantify the bowstringing effect induced after CTR and A1 pulley release and the differences between open and percutaneous techniques. However, the observation in one specimen needs to be confirmed by studying more specimens allowing a statistical analysis.

Although the decrease of FPL excursion with long finger extension could be explained by intertendinous connections between FLP and long finger flexor tendons, it seems more difficult to explain how the CTR makes this effect of long finger extension disappear. Further 3D kinematic and anatomic analysis on more specimens should be performed to better understand the underlying mechanism.

The 3D kinematic model proposed in this article will be able not only to compare new percutaneous procedures in terms of efficiency, possible iatrogenic lesions, and importance of postoperative bowstringing but also to bring additional information that could help to answer remaining questions about the link between CTR and preoperative and postoperative TF onset. Another information that could be also obtained is the evaluation of the relationship between long finger's flexor tendons and FPL before and after CTR to better understand

the modification of the distribution of TF onset after CTR when compared with isolated TF distribution.

SUMMARY

Improvement of sonography imaging and its use in an interventional manner gave birth to a promising new kind of minimally invasive hand surgery. CTR and TF release are procedures more and more performed using these new percutaneous sonographically guided techniques. Clinical studies are still scarce and heterogeneous. Biomechanical studies will help in precisely demonstrating the real advantages of these minimally invasive approaches. Questions about the bowstringing and its consequences on hand function as well as its role in the onset of TF after CTR are still debated. This article proposes an original biomechanical model that could help to asses these new procedures as well as try to answer still remaining questions.

ACKNOWLEDGMENTS

The authors gratefully acknowledge the assistance of Prof. Frédéric Schuind in conception of the presented study and in the writing of the present paper.

SUPPLEMENTARY DATA

Supplementary data related to this article can be found online at https://doi.org/10.1016/j.hcl.2021.08.010.

REFERENCES

1. Koenig RW, Schmidt TE, Heinen CP, et al. Intraoperative high-resolution ultrasound: a new technique in the management of peripheral nerve disorders. J Neurosurg 2011;114(2):514–21.
2. Yamamoto M, Kurimoto S, Okui N, et al. Sonography-assisted arthroscopic resection of volar wrist Ganglia: a new technique. Arthrosc Tech 2012;1(1):e31–5.
3. Chern TC, Jou IM, Yen SH, et al. Cadaver study of sonographically assisted percutaneous release of A1 pulley. Plast Reconstr Surg 2005;115:811–22.
4. Nakamichi K, Tachibana S. Ultrasonographically assisted carpal tunnel release. J Hand Surg Am 1997;22(5):853–62.
5. Lorthioir J Jr. Surgical treatment of trigger-finger by a subcutaneous method. J Bone Joint Surg Am 1958;40-A(4):793–5.
6. Rajeswaran G, Lee JC, Eckersley R, et al. Ultrasound-guided percutaneous release of the annular pulley in trigger digit. EurRadiol 2009;19(9):2232–7.
7. Rojo-Manaute JM, Rodríguez-Maruri G, Capa-Grasa A, et al. Sonographically guided intrasheath percutaneous release of the first annular pulley for trigger digits, part 1: clinical efficacy and safety. J Ultrasound Med 2012;31(3):417–24.
8. Rowe NM, Michaels J, Soltanian H, et al. Sonographically guided percutaneous carpal tunnel release: an anatomic and cadaveric study. Ann Plast Surg 2005;55(1):52–6.
9. Markison RE. A Percutaneous ultrasound-guided MANOS carpal tunnel release technique. Hand (N Y) 2013;8(4):445–9.
10. Chern TC, Wu KC, Huang LW, et al. A cadaveric and preliminaryclinical study of ultrasonographically assisted percutaneous carpal tunnel release. Ultrasound Med Biol 2014;40(8):1819–26.
11. Guo D, Guo D, Guo J, et al. A cadaveric study for the improvement of thread carpal tunnel release. J Hand Surg Am 2016;41(10):e351–7.
12. Petrover D, Silvera J, De Baere T, et al. Percutaneous ultrasound-guided carpal tunnel release: study upon clinical efficacy and safety. Cardiovasc Intervent Radiol 2017;40(4):568–75.
13. Kiritsis PG, Kline SC. Biomechanical changes after carpal tunnel release: a cadaveric model for comparing open, endoscopic, and step-cut lengthening techniques. J Hand Surg Am 1995;20(2):173–80.
14. Hamman J, Ali A, Phillips C, et al. A biomechanical study of the flexor digitorum superficialis: effects of digital pulley excision and loss of the flexor digitorum profundus. J Hand Surg Am 1997;22(2):328–35.
15. Hombal JW, Owen R. Carpal tunnel decompression and trigger digits. Hand 1970;2(2):192–6.
16. Zhang D, Collins J, Earp BE, et al. Relationship of carpal tunnel release and new onset trigger finger. J Hand Surg Am 2019;44(1):28–34.
17. Goshtasby PH, Wheeler DR, Moy OJ. Risk factors for trigger finger occurrence after carpal tunnel release. Hand Surg 2010;15(2):81–7.
18. Lee SK, Bae KW, Choy WS. The relationship of trigger finger and flexor tendon volar migration after carpal tunnel release. J Hand Surg Eur 2014;39(7):694–8.
19. Grandizio LC, Beck JD, Rutter MR, et al. The incidence of trigger digit after carpal tunnel release in diabetic and nondiabetic patients. J Hand Surg Am 2014;39(2):280–5.
20. An KN, Takahashi K, Harrigan TP, et al. Determination of muscle orientations and moment arms. J Biomech Eng 1984;106(3):280–2.
21. Lu SC, Yang TH, Kuo LC, et al. Effects of different extents of pulley release on tendon excursion efficiency and tendon moment arms. J Orthop Res 2015;33(2):224–8.
22. Hoang D, Lin AC, Essilfie A, et al. Evaluation of percutaneous first annular pulley release: efficacy and complications in a perfused cadaveric study. J Hand Surg Am 2016;41(7):e165–73.
23. Sobczak S, Rotsaert P, Vancabeke M, et al. Effects of proximal row carpectomy on wrist biomechanics: a cadaveric study. Clin Biomech (Bristol, Avon) 2011;26(7):718–24.
24. Merriaux P, Dupuis Y, Boutteau R, et al. A Study of Vicon System Positioning Performance. Sensors (Basel) 2017;17(7):1591.
25. Eichelberger P, Ferraro M, Minder U, et al. Analysis of accuracy in optical motion capture - A protocol for laboratory setup evaluation. J Biomech 2016;49(10):2085–8.

Volar Ganglion Cyst and Echo-Guided Assistance for the Arthroscopic Removal

Luc Van Overstraeten, MD, PhD[a,b,*], Emmanuel Jacques Camus, MD, PhD[c], Fabian Moungondo, MD, PhD[a], Frédéric Schuind, MD, PhD[a]

KEYWORDS

• Sonographically • Ganglion • Volar • Arthroscopy • Resection

KEY POINTS

- The wrist ganglion cyst is to be traited only when it's unconfortable.
- The wrist ganglion cyst recurs whatever the treatment.
- Arthroscopic resection of the wrist ganglion cyst reduces the risk of recurence.
- The volar ganglion cyst is located in the immediate proximity of the radial artery, the Flexor Pollicis Longus tendon and the median nerve.
- Echo-guided assistance reduces the risk of complications of volar ganglion cyst arthroscopic resection due to damage to these neighboring structures.

 Video content accompanies this article at http://www.hand.theclinics.com.

INTRODUCTION

The ganglion of the wrist is one of the most encountered hand surgery disease but whose prognosis is the least certain.

There seems to be a consensus regarding non-uncomfortable ganglions toward therapeutic abstention. Symptomatic wrist ganglions are usually treated conservatively as first-line treatment. When their volume Is sufficient, puncture infiltration leads to 50% permanent disappearance.

For occult ganglion cysts or recurrences of medical treatments, surgical resection is proposed, leading, depending on the series, to a recurrence in 6% to 59% of cases.[1] The literature is full of iatrogenic complications publications ranging from tendon or nerve damage to carpal instability.[2]

Arthroscopy offers a very different therapeutic methodology. First, it allows an inventory of the ligaments and cartilage. Then it aims to remove the ganglion from its pedicle.

Volar ganglions are close to the radial artery, the flexor pollicis longus (FPL) tendon, and even the median nerve. Ultrasonography combined with arthroscopy offers incomparable safety for the resection of volar ganglions.

EPIDEMIOLOGY

The ganglions constitute the most common tumors of the hand and wrist region, with a high incidence and prevalence. Ganglions occur more frequently in women (in the ratio of 3:1), between the second and fourth decades.[1] About 60% to 70% of the ganglions of the wrist are dorsal and

The authors have no conflict of interest to disclose.
[a] Orthopedic and Traumatologic, University Hospital Erasme, Brussels, Belgium; [b] Hand and Wrist Center, HFSU, AO Foundation, Tournai, Belgium; [c] Department of Orthopaedic and Traumatologic Surgery, University Clinical Center, Polyclinic Val de Sambre, Maubeuge, France
* Corresponding author.
E-mail address: Luc.van.overstraeten@skynet.be

Hand Clin 38 (2022) 101–107
https://doi.org/10.1016/j.hcl.2021.08.011
0749-0712/22/© 2021 Elsevier Inc. All rights reserved.

Table 1
Etiopathogenesis of wrist ganglion cyst

			Etiopathogenic Theories
1	1746	Eller	Herniation
	2008	Pliefke et al,[5] 2008	One-way valve mechanism
2	1926	Carp and Stout,[29] 1928	Rent theory: mucinous degeneration of connective tissue secondary to chronic damage
	1989	Watson et al,[11] 1989	Consequence of ligament injuries around the scaphoid
	2016	Van Overstraeten et al,[12] 2013	2d stage of DCSS lesion
3			Extra-articular mucoid degeneration
4			Result of continuous microinjuries to the capsular and ligamentous structure; stimulation of fibroblasts to produce hyaluronic acid

communicate with the joint by means of a pedicle; 13% to 20% of the ganglions are volar, arising via a pedicle from the radioscaphoid/scapholunate interval, scaphotrapezial joint, or the metacarpotrapezial joint, in that order of frequency.[3] Another 10% of the ganglions originate from a flexor tendon sheath.[4]

ETIOPATHOGENESIS

Little is known about the pathomechanism of the ganglion cyst formation. Several theories confront each other (**Table 1**).

The first suggests that the ganglion cyst would result from a herniation of the capsular synovial tissue. The cyst fluid that arises from the joint is pumped into the cyst via a 1-way valve mechanism. Microscopically, the pedicle contains a tortuous lumen, connecting the cyst to the underlying joint.[5,6] The presence of this connection is suspected with the demonstration of arthrographic intra-articular contrast opacification from the radiocarpal joint into the ganglion in 44% (dorsal ganglion) and 85% (volar ganglion) of patients. As contrast does not seem to travel from the cyst into the joint, a 1-way valve mechanism has been postulated.[7,8] Such a 1-way valve is thought to be formed by the number of small "microcysts" present in the tissue surrounding the pedicle. These "microcysts" communicate with the primary ganglion and are thought to be part of the tortuous pedicle lumen, connecting the cyst to the joint, and, in the process, creating the 1-way valve mechanism.[9] However, there is not synovial lining of the cyst wall, and the cyst fluid also has a different composition than intra-articular synovial fluid.[4,10]

The capsular rent theory is based on the assumption that injuries to the wrist joint lead to damage resulting in leakage of synovial fluid in the periarticular tissue. In support of this "capsular rent" theory, some investigators have postulated that preexisting joint pathology (periscaphoid ligamentous injury, etc.) is the underlying cause of rent/cyst formation. Joint abnormalities are thought to lead to altered biomechanics, eventual weakening of the capsule, and finally leakage of fluid and cyst formation. However, despite arthroscopic findings confirming the presence of intra-articular joint pathology in 50% of patients with ganglion, no correlation between this pathologic condition and postoperative ganglion recurrence can be demonstrated. This lack of correlation leads some investigators to conclude that intra-articular pathology is not the inciting event in the "rent" theory of ganglion formation. Watson and colleagues[11] suggested in a study of 1989 that a ganglion was caused by an underlying ligament injury around the scaphoid. However, the hypothesis that ligament pathology would be the cause of the formation of a ganglion remains controversial. The dorsal capsuloscapholunate septum (DCSS), a ligamentary structure constituting the scapholunate complex (SC), which extends from the dorsoradial part of the interfosseal ridge of the distal radius to the dorsal part of the scapholunate ligament and the proximal part of the dorsal intercarpal ligament and which would play a role of predynamic scapholunate stabilizer, presents in its first lesion stage microinjuries corresponding to occult microcysts.[12–14]

A third theory speculates that an extra-articular degenerative process (mucoid degeneration) would be the cause of both the formation of the ganglion and its direct connection to the joint.[4,10]

A fourth theory states that persistent irritation of the joint would incite the mesenchymal cells to the secretion of mucin. Small accumulations of mucin form the cyst around which a pseudocapsule develops without synovial alignment.[4] Alternatively, joint stress may lead to mucoid degeneration of adjacent extra-articular connective tissue with subsequent fluid accumulation and eventual ganglion formation. This theory holds that the cyst and pedicle form a direct connection to the joint only after the creation of the ganglion cyst.

DIAGNOSTIC METHODOLOGY: CLINICAL AND PARACLINICAL EXAMINATIONS
Clinical Examination

Ganglion cysts of the wrist come in 2 different forms: they can be easily visible or occult.

Often, the ganglion cyst appears as a single or multilocular nodular renitent swelling. Palmar cysts fill the pulse gutter without ever compressing the radial artery. Nevertheless, the clinical semiology of ganglion cysts requires a control of the permeability of the radial and ulnar arteries (Allen test). If visible, cysts are rarely painful during palpation. The mobility of the wrist is often normal. The discomfort can be painful and/or esthetic.

However, regularly, no tumor is palpable, but the patient describes a mechanical pain punctuated by the extreme amplitudes of mobilization. Ligament testing awakens a pain on the radioscaphocapitate ligament by a painful Watson maneuver but without a clunk. Grip strength may be reduced.

Paraclinic Examinations

Radiography
The standard wrist radiograph is essential in every assessment of wrist pain; it helps to rule out intraosseous injury, joint pinching, radiolucent formation in the soft tissues, or changes in interosseous relationships that indicate static instability.

Sonography
Ultrasonography is the gold standard for diagnosing a wrist ganglion cyst. The characteristic anechoic appearance of its mucoid content, its sharp and rounded limits, and the absence of vascular formation make its diagnosis all the easier the larger the volume. However, sometimes the size of the lesion is smaller than the discriminative capacity of the examination.

Arthro-CT
According to Moser, an arthro-CT (computed tomography) remains the gold standard for diagnosing a scapholunate interosseous ligament (SLIOL) injury. This is particularly true for documenting the transfixing or nontransfixing lesions of the dorsal part of the SLIOL in cross sections.[15] Sagittal sections sometimes show tiny millimeter-sized opacifications on the anterior surface of the distal metaphysis of the radius, in the area of

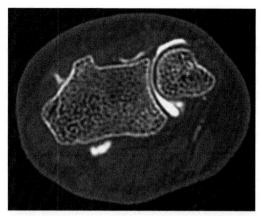

Fig. 1. Arthro-CT of a left wrist: transversal section showing an occult microcyst at the insertion of the RSC and LRL.

insertion of the radiosaphocapitate (RSC) and long radiolunate (LRL) ligaments, compatible with occult ganglion cysts. The inframillimetric thin sections of the examination improve discrimination **(Fig. 1)**.

MRI
MRI has recently been able, particularly after Shahabpour and colleagues' work, to document extrinsic ligaments and their injuries. The use of specific incidences in 3D reconstruction allows to obtain millimetric cuts that improve discrimination and refine the diagnosis of occult cysts and their relationship with certain extrinsic ligament injuries, constituent elements of the SC[16,17] **(Fig. 2)**.

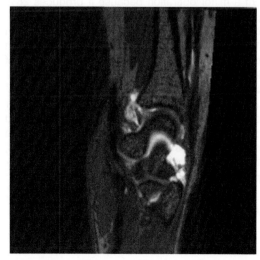

Fig. 2. MRI—sagittal view: occult ganglion cyst with hypersignal of RSC.

TREATMENT
Conservative Treatment

There seems to be a consensus in the world of hand surgeons concerning the management of wrist ganglion cysts: "Only treat annoying ganglions!" or "Do not turn an asymptomatic ganglion into a painful ganglion!" Depending on the series, the recurrence rate of ganglion cysts is between 6% and 59%, depending on whether it follows an arthroscopic resection or a puncture aspiration.[18] Therefore, the first-line treatment remains the blind puncture of the cyst immediately followed by an injection of corticoid deposits. The aseptic conditions must be surgical. The gauge of the puncture needles will be inversely proportional to the fluidity of the mucoid liquid, and it varies from 18 to 21. Generally, the thickness of the liquid is proportional to the age of the ganglion cyst. Personally, we prefer to use betamethasone rather than methylprednisolone as a corticoid deposit.

Sonography-Guided Puncture and Infiltration

Ultrasound guidance does not seem to improve the prognosis.[18] Nevertheless, it obviously helps to aspirate small volume ganglion cysts; it prevents hematomas linked to the puncture of volar ganglions, but does not improve the recurrence rate, which remains at 66% in an average period of 9 months.[19]

Open Resection

Surgical resection of dorsal ganglion cysts requires complete removal of all the cyst connections to the SC structures.[6] Surgical resection is not a minor operation because it produces 28% persistent pain, limitation of function, dissatisfaction, or recurrence.[20,21] The recurrence occurs in 10% of cases and is not significantly different in dorsal or palmar resections.[20] There are risks of injury of radial artery branches (16%) (with sometimes a pseudoaneurysm) or neurapraxia (4%).[21] The risk of scapholunate destabilization after open dorsal ganglion excision is an expected concern because SC components could be resected with the ganglion cyst. Nevertheless, this risk is not confirmed by the literature, which reports only a few isolated cases.[22,23]

ARTHROSCOPIC RESECTION

The arthroscopy is performed under axillary plexus anesthesia, under pneumatic tourniquet, with 6-kg zenital traction, using "Chinese" finger traps, with a brachial counterbearing.

A 2.4-mm arthroscope with 30° angulation is used through 2 radiocarpal (3-4) and (4-5) portals and 2 radial and ulnar midcarpal and portals. The arthroscopy performed by dry procedure begins with an assessment of the ligaments and cartilage. The scapholunate and lunotriquetral stability is checked according to the EWAS (European Wrist Arthroscopy Society) classification,[24] and then each accessible extrinsic ligament and the DCSS are evaluated by means of a specific probe test.[12,13,25] The cartilage is also assessed according to Outerbridge's modified classification.[26] Finally, the triangular fibrocartilaginous complex is tested on its foveal and peripheral attachments.

At the dorsal side, the location of the ganglion cyst is most often determined by the bulging of the joint caused by pressure or pinching of the cyst. The bulge is best seen at the level of the dorsal capsule, sometimes with a central translucency. Cystic puncture with an 18-gauge needle confirms this location. Capsular resection with a 2.0- or 3.0-mm arthroscopic shaver can then begin until the common extensor tendons of the fingers are visualized. Sometimes the cyst is very small and pedicles on a microlesion of the DCSS. Arthroscopic debridement should then only concern the cystic lesion, respecting the other arches of the DCSS, and ensuring that the scapholunar space remains closed. Cystic mucoid injection with methylene blue is described, but we have never used it because joint contamination by the dye quickly makes the dry procedure impossible.

The palmar ganglion cyst most often pediculates at the level of the interligamentous sulcus, between the RSC and the LRL ligaments. In this case, the opening of the sulcus by the introduction of the probe very often causes viscous synovial jelly to flow into the joint from the cyst. The debridement of the cystic pedicle is performed with the shaver without penetrating into the volar extra-articular soft tissues beyond 3 to 4 mm so as not to cause injury to the FPL tendon or the radial artery. The risk of radial artery injury with this arthroscopic procedure is lesser (4%) than with volar ganglion open resection.[21]

The ganglion cyst can pedicle into the radioscapholunate (RSL) ligament or between this RSL ligament and the short radiolunate ligament. The procedure remains the same: debridement of the pedicle with the shaver by pressing the cyst from the outside.

RECONSTRUCTIVE REINFORCEMENT

In 2013, in an unpublished lecture, Gustavo Mantovani suggested, to treat recurrence of dorsal

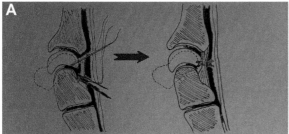
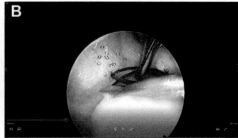

Fig. 3. Mathoulin's dorsal capsuloligamentary reinforcement. (*A*) Passage of the suture from the radiocarpal to the mediocarpal suture node. (*B*) Midcarpal view of the both needles and sutures.

arthrosynovial cyst after arthroscopic resection, that a Mathoulin's dorsal capsuloligamentary reinforcement should be performed[27] (**Fig. 3**). This procedure is in fact a reconstruction of the DCSS. This reconstruction is also suggested for the primary treatment of dorsal cysts with predynamic scapholunate instability.

SONOGRAPHICALLY GUIDED RESECTION OF VOLAR GANGLION CYST OF THE WRIST

In recent years, ultrasonography has been introduced into surgical consultations and then quite rapidly into surgical programs. Ultrasonography guides specialists daily to perform plexus anesthesia. Percutaneous ultrasound-guided surgery has now become a regular practice to treat the trigger finger or the carpal tunnel.

To secure the arthroscopic resection of palmar arthrosynovial cysts in its intimate relationship with the radial artery, the FPL tendon, and the median nerve, ultrasonography is nowadays systematically associated with the arthroscopic procedure described earlier.

The operation is done without tourniquet. A high-frequency linear array transducer of 12 MHz frequency (GE Healthcare LOGIQ *e,* General Electric Company, USA) covered by a sterile drape is used by an assisting surgeon during the wrist arthroscopy. The surgeon who performs the arthroscopy, experienced in hand surgery and sonography, directs the use of sonography. The arthroscope and sonography screens are placed beyond the patient so that they can be easily viewed by the surgeon (**Fig. 4**).

After the arthroscopic testing time and precise localization of the ganglion pedicle, the arthroscope is introduced through 4-5 portal and then maintained by the surgical assistant. The shaver introduced through 3-4 portal is held by the surgeon's dominant hand, while he manipulates with the other hand the ultrasound probe placed on the distal relief of the flexor carpi radialis tendon

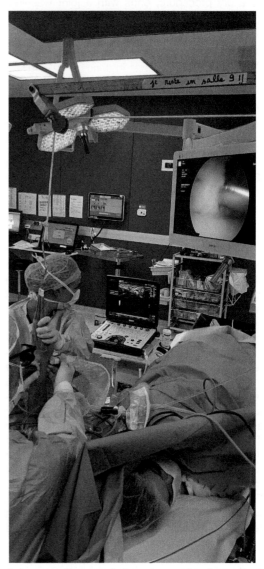

Fig. 4. Installation of the sonographically assisted arthroscopic resection procedure. Sonographic and arthroscopic screens.

and the radial pulse zone. The head of the shaver must never disappear completely into the interligamentous sulcus, and the ultrasound must keep the radial artery on screen at all times. The sulcus is widely opened by separating the fibers of the RSC and LRL ligaments rather than resecting them. By digital pressure, the cyst is completely drained into the joint. It is useless, and moreover strongly discouraged, to introduce the shaver completely into the ganglion pouch, because in this case, ultrasound control cannot guarantee that a recurrent small arterial branch lesion will be avoided and therefore a zero risk of hematoma or pseudoaneurysm.

The procedure, which was previously performed as a dry procedure, ends with a joint washing, closure of the arthroscopic portals, and a dressing. Cast immobilization is not systematic.

DISCUSSION

A 2015 meta-analysis of 35 studies and 2239 ganglions reports that arthroscopic resection is significantly more effective and safe than open resection. Indeed, the recurrence and complication rates are significantly lower for arthroscopic resection (6% and 4%, respectively) than for open resection (21% and 14%). The study reports a recurrence rate of 59% after puncture infiltration.[17]

In a series of 42 patients operated on by sonography-guided arthroscopic excision of an arthrosynovial cyst (26 dorsal and 16 volar), Yamamoto and colleagues[28] reported no recurrence of volar ganglion and concluded that "the use of sonography-guided arthroscopic ganglion excision is better for treating volar wrist ganglion than dorsal wrist ganglion." This superior interest in the use of sonography-guided arthroscopic excision for volar cysts could be justified by the fact that open excision would make no significant difference in recurrence according to the volar or dorsal situation of the resected ganglion.[20] However, it should be remembered that the primary interest of echo guidance remains to ensure the integrity of vascular structures that are highly threatened by the shaver if blindly used. Moreover, it is also possible that the difference in recurrence is linked more to the etiopathogenic difference of the volar and dorsal cysts than to the technique used to resect them. From this point of view, dorsal shaving could aggravate certain lesions of the DCSS rather than respecting the scapholunar stabilizer, and therefore could explain a higher recurrence rate.

Yamamoto and colleagues[28] also reported technical difficulties to perform sonography-guided arthroscopic excision of dorsal ganglion cysts. Because dorsal portals are used for arthroscopy,

the sonography transducer can impede the shaver for dorsal wrist ganglion. In some cases of dorsal wrist ganglions, it is difficult to use both sonography and arthroscopy at the same time.[28] However, for these investigators, in cases of volar wrist ganglion, sonography was always effective to visualize the relationship of the shaver, ganglion, and surrounding structures.[28] Therefore, the surgeon could use the shaver until making the path from joint to ganglion without concern for a neurovascular or tendon injury.

SUMMARY

The treatment of wrist ganglion cysts is indicated only when they are troublesome. The treatment is primarily conservative. Arthroscopic resection limits the risk of recurrence. Joint sonography secures the resection of volar ganglion cysts.

CLINICS CARE POINTS

- Sonographic guidance is not used for arthroscopic resection of dorsal ganglion cyst.
- During echo-guided arthroscopic resection of volar ganglion cyst, the assisting surgeon holds the arthroscope while the surgeon holds the ultrasound probe.
- The tip of the shaver should be sonographically checked away from arterial elements at all times.
- The first step in arthroscopic testing is the identification of the ganglion cyst articular opening usually in the sulcus between the Radio-Scapho-Capitatum ligament en the Long-Radio-Lunate ligament.
- It is not necessary to remove the entire cystic sac. It is mainly the ganglion pedicle that need to be resected.

SUPPLEMENTARY DATA

Supplementary data to this article can be found online at https://doi.org/10.1016/j.hcl.2021.08.011.

REFERENCES

1. Fernandes CH, Meirelles LM, Raduan Neto J, et al. Arthroscopic resection of dorsal wrist ganglion: results and rate of recurrence over a minimum follow-up of 4 years. Hand (N Y). 2019;14(2):236–41.

2. Cooper AR, Elfar JC. Extensor tendon lacerations from arthroscopic excision of dorsal wrist ganglion: case report. J Hand Surg Am 2013;38(10):1957–9.

3. Greendyke SD, Wilson M, Shepler TR. Anterior wrist ganglia from the scaphotrapezial joint. J Hand Surg Am 1992;17(3):487–90.

4. Gude W, Morelli V. Ganglion cysts of the wrist: pathofysiology, clinical picture, and management. Curr Rev Musculoskelet Med 2008;1(3–4):205–11.

5. Pliefke J, Stengel D, Rademacher G, et al. Diagnostic accuracy of plain radiographs and cineradiography in diagnosing traumatic scapholunate dissociation. Skeletal Radiol 2008;37(2):139–45.

6. Angelides AC, Wallace PF. The dorsal ganglion of the wrist: its pathogenesis, gross and microscopic anatomy, and surgical treatment. J Hand Surg Am 1976;1(3):228–35.

7. Linscheid RL, Dobyns JH, Beabout JW, et al. Traumatic instability of the wrist.Diagnosis, classification, and pathomechanics. J Bone Joint Surg Am 1972; 54(8):1612–32.

8. Garcia-Elias M, LluchAL. Wrist Instabilities, misalignments, and dislocations. In: Wolfe SW, Hotchkiss RN, Pederson WC, et al, editors. Green's operative Surgery. 7th edition. Philadelphia: Elsevier; 2017. p. 426–78.

9. Gilula LA, Destouet JM, Weeks PM, et al. Roentgenographic diagnosis of the painful wrist. Clin Orthop Relat Res 1984;187:52–64.

10. Dias JJ, Dhukaram V, Kumar P. The natural history of untreated dorsal wrist ganglia and patient reported outcome 6 years after intervention. J Hand Surg Eur 2007;32(5):502–8.

11. Watson HK, Rogers WD, Ashmead D. Reevaluation of the cause of the wrist ganglion. J Hand Surg Am 1989;14(5):812–7.

12. Van Overstraeten L, Camus EJ, Wahegaonkar A, et al. Anatomical description of the dorsal capsuloscapholunate septum (DCSS)-arthroscopic staging of scapholunate instability after DCSS sectioning. J Wrist Surg 2013;2(2):149–54.

13. Van Overstraeten L, Camus EJ. Arthroscopic classification of the lesions of the dorsal capsuloscapholunate septum (DCSS) of the wrist. Tech Hand Up Extrem Surg 2016;20(3):125–8.

14. Garret J, Facca S, Bordet B, et al. Dorsal mucoid cyst of the wrist: Pathology and epidemiology. Rev Chir Orthop Traum 2017;103(8):S179–84.

15. Moser T, Dosch JC, Moussaoui A, et al. Multidetector CT arthrography of the wrist joint: how to do it. Radiographics 2008;(28):787–800.

16. Shahabpour M, Van Overstraeten L, Ceuterick P, et al. Pathology of extrinsic ligaments: a pictorial essay. Semin Musculo Skelet Radiol 2012;(16):115–28.

17. Shahabpour M, De Maeseneer M, Pouders C, et al. MR imaging of normal extrinsic wrist ligaments using thin slices with clinical and surgical correlation. Eur J Radiol 2011;(77):196–201.

18. Head L, Gencarelli JR, Allen M, et al. Wrist ganglion treatment: systematic review and meta-analysis. J Hand Surg Am 2015;40(3):546–53.e8.

19. Gitto S, Lee SC, Miller TT. Ultrasound-guided percutaneous treatment of volar radiocarpal ganglion cysts: Safety and efficacy. J Clin Ultrasound 2019; 47(6):339–44.

20. Faithfull DK, Seeto BG. The simple wrist ganglion–more than a minor surgical procedure? Hand Surg 2000 Dec;5(2):139–43.

21. Rocchi L, Canal A, Fanfani F, et al. Articular ganglia of the volar aspect of the wrist: arthroscopic resection compared with open excision. A prospective randomised study. Scand J Plast Reconstr Surg Hand Surg 2008;42(5):253–9.

22. Dermon A, Kapetanakis S, Fiska A, et al. Ganglionectomy without repairing the bursal defect: long-term results in a series of 124 wrist ganglia. Clin Orthop Surg 2011;3(2):152–6.

23. Duncan KH, Lewis RC Jr. Scapholunate instability following ganglion cyst excision. A case report. Clin Orthop Relat Res 1988 Mar;(228):250–3.

24. Messina JC, Van Overstraeten L, Luchetti R, et al. The EWAS classification of scapholunate tears: an anatomical arthroscopic study. J Wrist Surg 2013;(2):105–9.

25. Van Overstraeten L, Camus E. A systematic method of arthroscopic testing of extrinsic carpal ligaments: implication in carpal stability. Tech Hand Surg 2013;(17).202–6.

26. Van Overstraeten L, Camus EJ. Arthroscopic criteria for dating wrist sprains. Chir Main 2012;(31):171–5.

27. Wahegaonkar AL, Mathoulin CL. Arthroscopic dorsal capsulo-ligamentous repair in the treatment of chronic scapho-lunate ligament tears. J Wrist Surg 2013;(2):141–8.

28. Yamamoto M, Kurimoto S, Iwatsuki K, et al. Sonography-guided arthroscopic excision is more effective for treating volar wrist ganglion than dorsal wrist ganglion. Acta Orthop Belg 2018;84(1):78–83.

29. Carp L, Stout AP. A study of ganglion. Surg Gynec Obstet 1928;47:460–8.

Using Ultrasonography During the Fixation of Distal Radius and Finger Fractures

Jean Michel Cognet, MD[a],*, François Bauzou, MD[b], Pascal Louis, MD[a], Olivier Mares, MD[b]

KEYWORDS

- Distal radius • Finger fracture • Ultrasound • Ultrasonography

KEY POINTS

- Ultrasonography (US) is a noninvasive examination modality that is devoid of risk, both for the patient and the surgeon.
- the operating time is reduced when US is used primarily, as it is much easier to manipulate than a fluoroscopy system.
- The superiority of US over radiographs for detecting overly long screws has been showed by some studies but must be emphazed by much larger scale studies.

INTRODUCTION

Assessing the reduction of a distal radius or finger fracture and the subsequent implant positioning typically requires an intraoperative check using fluoroscopy. But using fluoroscopy requires protective measures because of the resulting radiation. The risk level varies based on the patient, duration of exposure, and repetitive nature of certain procedures. In several countries, using a fluoroscopy system also requires an accreditation that must be renewed every 3 years through training.

Ultrasonography (US) is a noninvasive examination modality that is devoid of risk, both for the patient and the surgeon. US imaging expands the possibilities to the diagnosis of occult fractures and the evaluation of fracture reduction. The costs of purchasing and maintaining US systems have greatly decreased in recent years, and no radiation protective measures are required during use. We have combined this diagnostic ability with an assessment of the fixation of distal radius, metacarpal, and phalangeal fractures.

EQUIPMENT NEEDED

We currently use a Samsung system (HS 40) consisting of a standard probe (3–16 MHz) and a finger-specific probe (17–18 MHz). Although it is possible to use a lower-grade system (4–12 MHz probe), the image quality will be lower but still acceptable for checking distal radius and finger fractures (**Fig. 1**).

Because the probe is not sterile, we use protective sleeves such as the ones used for arthroscopy. We recommend using an inner sleeve (provided with the single-use kit) and combining it with an arthroscopy sleeve (**Fig. 2**). Sterile gel is placed on the probe before applying the first sleeve, then the second sleeve is used to cover the entire length of the probe's cable (**Figs. 3–5**).

Conflict of Interests: none.
[a] SOS Mains Champagne Ardenne, Médipôle, 1 rue Jules Méline, Bezannes 51430, France; [b] Service de Chirurgie Orthopédique et Traumatologique, Centre Hospitalo-Universitaire Carémeau, 4 Rue du Professeur Robert Debré, Nîmes 30029, France
* Corresponding author.
E-mail address: jmrc@free.fr

hand.theclinics.com

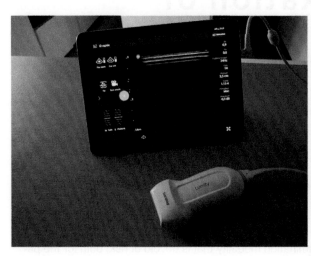
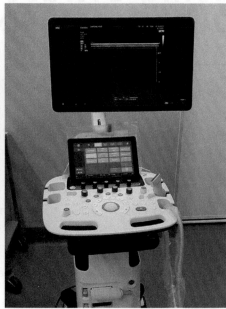

Fig. 1. A Philips 4 to 12 MHz probe coupled with an Android tablet (*left*) and a SAMSUNG HS 40 US system with 3 to 16 MHz probe (*right*).

Procedures

The patient is positioned supine, with a tourniquet at the base of the arm and the arm on an arm board; the fluoroscopy system is turned on, facing the surgeon. The US probe rests on the operating table, and the device is located at the end of the arm board (see **Figs. 4** and **5**).

During one's early cases, it may be helpful to do a control US scan to set the gain and depth. After doing a few procedures with the same system,

these parameters will stay the same. The gain is typically set at 60 and the depth at 3.5 cm for distal radius fractures and 1.5 cm from phalangeal/metacarpal fractures. Many systems allow a user's preferred settings to be stored so they can be reused each time.

DISTAL RADIUS FRACTURES

The procedure involves 3 steps, irrespective of the type of fixation:

- US detection of the fracture lines and comparison with preoperative radiographs
- Reduction and stabilization of fracture site
- Final fixation

Step 1: Ultrasonography Detection of the Fracture Lines and Comparison with Preoperative Radiographs

An initial scan is made to locate the fracture site and detect any changes in the anatomic landmarks (**Fig. 6**):

- Distal radioulnar joint on a transverse view (a)
- Lister's tubercle on a transverse view (b)
- Dorsal cortex of radius on a transverse view (c)
- Anterior curvature of radius to the watershed line on a sagittal view (d)
- Posterior cortex of distal radius on sagittal view (e)

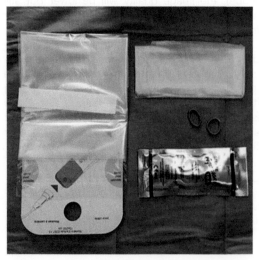

Fig. 2. Arthroscopy sleeve (*left*) and sleeve for US unit, elastics, and gel pocket (center from top to bottom).

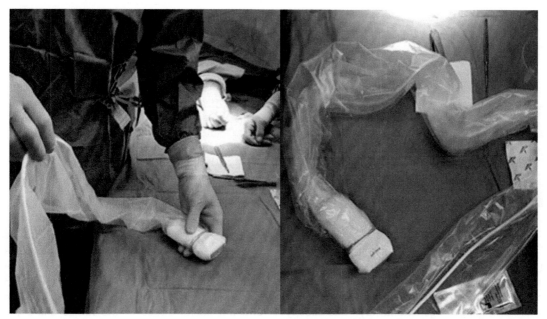

Fig. 3. Probe covered by an US sleeve (*left*) with an additional longer arthroscopy sleeve (*right*) that can cover the entire length of the cable.

The main landmarks are the anterior and posterior cortex of the distal radius. On a fracture with posterior tilt, the dorsal cortex is always modified and clearly visible. Loss of the anterior curvature is sometimes harder to detect on a dorsally displaced fracture. Transverse views of Lister tubercle and the diaphysis display an interesting elevator effect when done dynamically: sweeping the US probe over the dorsal side of the distal radius from proximal to distal will identify gradual elevation of the diaphysis up to Lister tubercle. In case of a dorsally displaced fracture, there is a sudden change in diameter from the diaphysis to the metaphysis of the radius; in some instances, there will be a double contour when the bones overlap.

Other structures are easy to pinpoint such as the pronator quadratus and the surrounding nerves, arteries, and tendons.

Step 2: Reduction and Stabilization of Fracture Site

The US step does not alter the fixation technique in any way. We typically use a locking plate designed specifically for distal radius fractures. However, although the fracture site is stabilized by the plate, we used the PY technique[1] to reduce the fracture site. Pinning can be done either before the plate is applied, after using US as a reference, or simply based on the preoperative radiographs. It is done by hand, without a motorized handpiece.

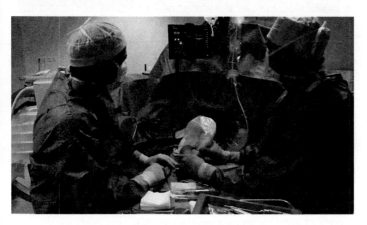

Fig. 4. Operating room set-up; the surgeon manipulates the probe, with the screen on the right beside the patient and the surgical assistant standing across from them.

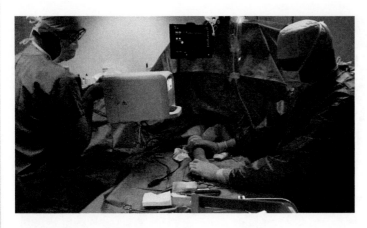

Fig. 5. Fluoroscopy can be paired with US when needed.

If the initial reduction is done first with K-wires, US images are then taken to check the reduction. The bone topography of the anterior cortex is clearly visible on US with much better definition than on images generated by fluoroscopy (**Fig. 7**). When the displacement is mainly posterior without a break in the anterior cortex, US imaging assesses the reduction of the posterior cortex, which is also clearly visible (**Fig. 8**).

In certain cases, excessive reduction can be observed on US even though it cannot be seen on fluoroscopy (**Fig. 9**).

The volar plate can be implanted through a Henry approach. A visual check of the fracture site is done to confirm the US images. The locking plate is set in its anterior position and held in place by a nonlocking screw placed in the oval slot. The plate's position is adjusted with the fingers relative to the watershed line and the lateral edges of the radius shaft; the preferred location is on the ulnar aspect of the radial diaphysis.

Another US image is taken at this point to verify the various anatomic landmarks and the elimination of any excessive reduction. Once the plate is in place, it is more difficult to see the anterior cortex on US; thus, the check revolves around Lister tubercle and the radial side of the distal radius. At this point, we look for dorsal cortical breach of the first screw.

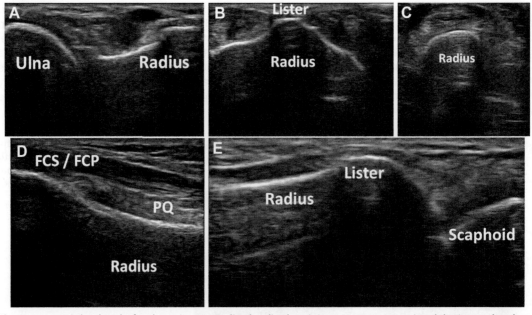

Fig. 6. Anatomic landmarks for the wrist on US: distal radioulnar joint on a transverse view (*A*), Lister tubercle on a transverse view (*B*), dorsal cortex of radius on a transverse view (*C*), anterior curvature of radius up to the watershed line on a sagittal view (*D*), posterior cortex of distal radius on a sagittal view (*E*).

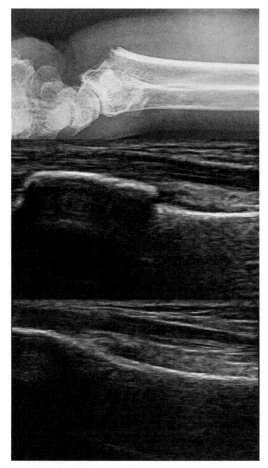

Fig. 7. US view of the reduction of the anterior cortex of the distal radius.

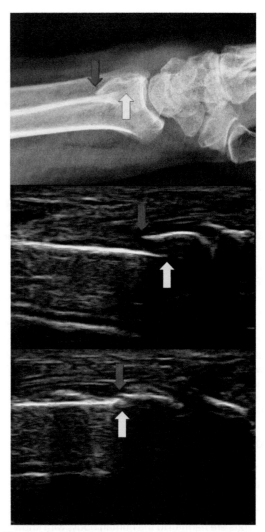

Fig. 8. US view of the reduction of the posterior cortex of the distal radius.

If there is a large displacement, US is used to identify the median nerve, check its integrity, and look for impingement by a bone splinter (**Figs. 10 and 11**); this is especially valuable when the patient presents with paresthesia in the territory of the median nerve.

Step 3: Final Fixation

If the surgeon is not certain whether the plate is in the correct position (too distal) or is concerned that a screw may be protruding inside the joint, a K-wire is pushed into the drilled hole and its exit point checked with US. Once the epiphyseal screws are in place, the surgeon moves the wrist to ensure there is no impingement with the implanted device (intraarticular projection of screw). The distal radioulnar joint also needs to be tested. We look at the dorsal cortex of the distal radius to see if a screw is sticking out (**Fig. 12**).

In a surgeon's early cases, we recommend pairing fluoroscopy checks with US checks at each step to confirm the fracture's reduction and the plate's correct positioning. One should start with simple, extraarticular fractures (eg, Pouteau/Colles). Later on, a surgeon can progress to using this technique with intraarticular fractures as long as it is combined with an arthroscopy assessment. In fact, it is impossible to view the intraarticular step off or subsidence if the fracture occurred in the central area of the scaphoid's or lunate's articular fossa.

PHALANGEAL AND METACARPAL FRACTURES

The principle is the same as for distal radius fractures: replace the fluoroscopy checks with US checks to reduce the patient's, surgeon's, and surgical team's exposure to radiation.

The US checks involve looking at the alignment of the cortices (because these are long bones) and

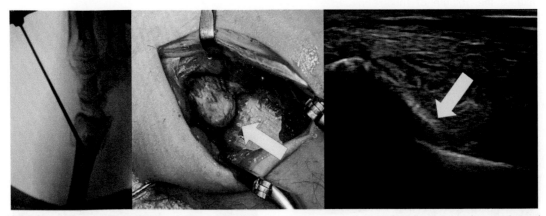

Fig. 9. This anterior overreduction is not visible on fluoroscopy but was detected with US; note the good match between the US image and the intraoperative appearance.

looking for device protrusion (screws, K-wires) (**Figs. 13** and **14**).

If doing open fracture fixation, US is used to look for screw protrusion. If doing percutaneous fracture fixation, US is used to verify the reduction of the fracture site and assess K-wire protrusion and its exit point. Planning is essential if we truly want to avoid using intraoperative fluoroscopy. If doing cross-pinning of a phalangeal fracture, it is important to define the desired path of the K-wires and trace it on the skin in both planes.

DISCUSSION

Intraoperative verification of fracture fixation requires the use of a radiography device in the operating room, and this provides an image of the fracture reduction and implants. However, radiographs are harmful to the human body, with known increased risks of skin cancer, especially in hand surgery, but also of thyroid cancer and cataracts.[2–4] In recent years, the introduction of mini C-arm systems designed for the extremities has reduced the risks related to radiographs but has not eliminated them.[5] Finding an alternative to radiographs during fracture fixation would be a positive step both for the patients and the surgical team.

There are currently no published articles that reported the possibility of doing US-guided distal radius fracture fixation. The existing studies describe verifying the reduction of distal radius fractures.[6–8] Conversely, studies have been done to compare fixation of a metacarpal facture with either fluoroscopy or US guidance.[9,10]

Ang and colleagues[6] reported their results of closed wrist fracture reduction on an emergency basis. By generating US images, the number of manipulations was reduced, and the reduction improved.

In 2014, Kodama and colleagues[7] compared 43 patients with a distal radius fracture that was reduced by US guidance to 57 patients who had their fracture reduced manually with or without fluoroscopy checks. The success of the reduction was the same in both groups.

More recently, Lau and colleagues[8] evaluated the contribution of US to the diagnosis and verification of reduction in patients with a distal radius fracture. They also determined how the person doing the US (radiologist or not) affected the result. Here again, US yielded results equal to that of radiography, independent of the operator.

Pediatricians have been using US to diagnose traumatic fractures for several years. The sensitivity of US is better than the sensitivity of radiographs for detecting fractures in children.[11–14] The specificity of US is better than the specificity of radiographs, at least for diagnosing fractures in children. Chen and Moore[12] found 14 false positives due to radiographs in a cohort of 110 children who had a nondisplaced fracture of both forearm bones.

In adults, US imaging is at the forefront when radiographs are not sufficient to make a diagnosis. This is the case for fatigue fractures where radiographs are normal early on, whereas US can reveal the changes needed to make a diagnosis.[15] Banal and colleagues[16] showed that the sensitivity of US was equal to that of MRI but that US was easier to schedule and cost substantially less. The availability of US and the miniaturization of the workstations have contributed to US being increasingly used in sports medicine.[17] A fracture could be diagnosed immediately after the injury occurs, even when there is no access to x-ray machine.

Several investigators contend that US diagnosis of fractures should be expanded to all bone traumas. Its relevance is supported in situations

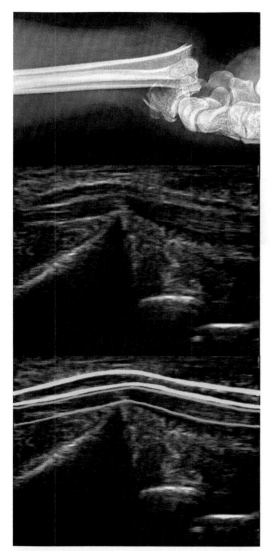

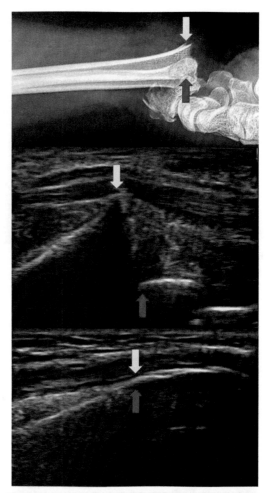

Fig. 11. Ultrasonography verification of reduction based on anterior cortex of distal radius; red arrow corresponds to proximal limit of distal fragment; yellow arrow corresponds to distal limit of proximal fragment. When the two arrows are lined up, the fracture is reduced.

Fig. 10. Extraarticular distal radius fracture with large displacement, the patient described having paresthesia in the median nerve territory. Sagittal US view before and after reduction showing the location of the flexor tendons (green) and the median nerve (yellow) relative to the fracture site: despite the large displacement, we can see that the median nerve is still protected by the flexor tendons.

where radiographs can be misleading, as in scaphoid fractures[18–20] or when screening for bone injuries in the emergency room.[21]

After demonstrating that US was reliable for analyzing and diagnosing fractures, the next step was real-time intraoperative verification of fracture reduction and implant positioning. When doing K-wire fixation, experienced surgeons can determine the percutaneous insertion point based on the preoperative imaging or directly with US guidance as described.[22]

However, US-guided plate fixation of a fracture has its challenges:

- Good positioning of the plate on the radius
- Verification of screw trajectory and exit point

Positioning of Plate on the Radius

The plate must be sufficiently distal so that the locking screws act as a strut on the articular surface. The further away the locking screws, the higher the risk of losing the reduction.[23] If the plate is too low, the risk of intraarticular screw penetration is high, as is the risk of flexor tendon injury, especially the flexor pollicis longus.[24,25] The plate must not extend beyond the distal border of the pronator quadratus, also known as the watershed line.

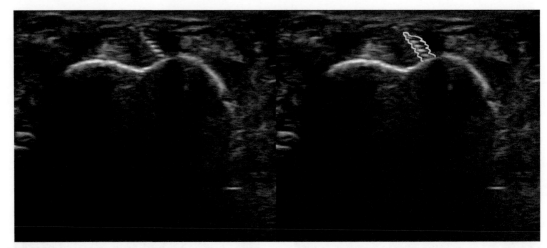

Fig. 12. Frontal view of the radial metaphysis where a screw protrudes beyond the cortex.

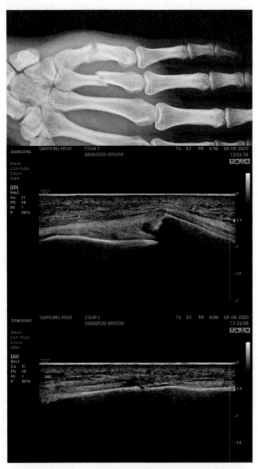

Fig. 13. Ideal view of the reduction of a displaced metacarpal fracture.

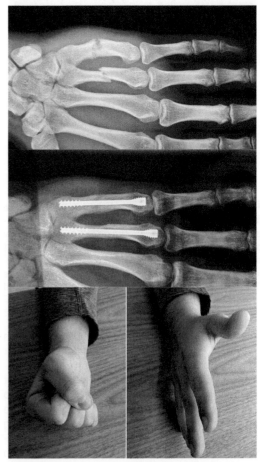

Fig. 14. Fixation was done using an intramedullary screw; clinical result at 3 months.

The plate must also be centered on the distal radius. This centering can be achieved by moving the plate manually using the ulnar side of the radius as a reference, which provides diaphyseal alignment. We did it this way each time and did not need to alter the plate's position after the fluoroscopy check.

Verification of Screw Trajectory and Exit Point

US can only show the bone's surface. Without radiographs, it is impossible to verify the screw's entry point visually and the exit point on the posterior cortex. The superiority of US over radiographs for detecting overly long screws has not been clearly demonstrated.[26,27] We believe the biggest risk is missing a screw whose tip protrudes inside the joint.

Fixation of Phalanges and Metacarpals

There are few published studies on US being used during the fixation of phalangeal and metacarpal fractures.[9,10] Studies comparing percutaneous pinning of metacarpal factures found similar results in terms of bone union and function. The only difference was the irradiation, which was lower in the US group. These articles seem to validate use of US as an alternative or supplement to fluoroscopy. Our experience in this area pushes us to continue using US imaging. But this requires a different strategy, with the need to further plan the procedure.

During the learning curve, irrespective of the type of fixation, the operating time is increased relative to a procedure done without US guidance. However, this increase is due to the double fluoroscopy and US checks being done more often. In the end, the operating time is reduced when US is used primarily, as it is much easier to manipulate than a fluoroscopy system.

US is a tool that can benefit both the patient and surgeon. Its harmlessness, the increasing quality of its images, and the decrease in the cost of US systems means that we should consider it as an alternative to daily use of radiographs.

CLINICS CARE POINTS

- the probe is not sterile, we use protective sleeves such as the ones used for arthroscopy.
- We recommend using an inner sleeve (provided with the single-use kit) and combining it with an arthroscopy sleeve.

- In certain cases, excessive reduction can be observed on US even though it cannot be seen on fluoroscopy.
- Once the plate is in place, it is more difficult to see the anterior cortex on US; thus, the check revolves around Lister tubercle and the radial side of the distal radius. At this point, we look for dorsal cortical breach of the first screw.

REFERENCES

1. Desmanet E. [Osteosynthesis in double elastic nailing of radial shortening osteotomy in Kienbock disease. Apropos of 4 cases]. Rev Chir Orthop Reparatrice Appar Mot 1996;82(4):327–30. L'osteosynthese par double embrochage souple des osteotomies de raccourcissement du radius pour maladie de Kienbock. A propos de 4 cas.
2. Chambers JA, Long JN. Radiation injury and the hand surgeon. J Hand Surg Am 2008;33(4):601–11.
3. Frazier TH, Richardson JB, Fabre VC, et al. Fluoroscopy-induced chronic radiation skin injury: a disease perhaps often overlooked. Arch Dermatol 2007;143(5):637–40.
4. Mastrangelo G, Fedeli U, Fadda E, et al. Increased cancer risk among surgeons in an orthopaedic hospital. Occup Med (Lond) 2005;55(6):498–500.
5. van Rappard JRM, Hummel WA, de Jong T, et al. A Comparison of Image Quality and Radiation Exposure Between the Mini C-Arm and the Standard C-Arm. Hand (N Y) 2018. https://doi.org/10.1177/1558944718770210. 1558944718770210.
6. Ang S-H, Lee S-W, Lam K-Y. Ultrasound-guided reduction of distal radius fractures. Am J Emerg Med 2010;28(9):1002–8.
7. Kodama N, Takemura Y, Ueba H, et al. Ultrasound-Assisted Closed Reduction of Distal Radius Fractures. J Hand Surg 2014;39(7):1287–94.
8. Lau BC, Robertson A, Motamedi D, et al. The Validity and Reliability of a Pocket-Sized Ultrasound to Diagnose Distal Radius Fracture and Assess Quality of Closed Reduction. J Hand Surg 2017;42(6):420–7.
9. Wang L, Wang X, Li W. [Effectiveness comparison between ultrasound-guided and C-arm-guided in closed reduction and pinning for treatment of metacarpophalangeal fractures]. Zhongguo Xiu Fu Chong Jian Wai Ke Za Zhi 2017;31(10):1179–83.
10. Shen S, Wang X, Fu Z. Value of Ultrasound-Guided Closed Reduction and Minimally Invasive Fixation in the Treatment of Metacarpal Fractures. J Ultrasound Med 2019;38(10):2659–66.
11. Ko C, Baird M, Close M, et al. The Diagnostic Accuracy of Ultrasound in Detecting Distal Radius Fractures in a Pediatric Population. Clin J Sport Med 2017. https://doi.org/10.1097/jsm.0000000000000547.

12. Chen L, Kim Y, Moore CL. Diagnosis and guided reduction of forearm fractures in children using bedside ultrasound. Pediatr Emerg Care 2007; 23(8):528–31.

13. Chaar-Alvarez FM, Warkentine F, Cross K, et al. Bedside ultrasound diagnosis of nonangulated distal forearm fractures in the pediatric emergency department. Pediatr Emerg Care 2011;27(11):1027–32.

14. Warkentine FH, Horowitz R, Pierce MC. The use of ultrasound to detect occult or unsuspected fractures in child abuse. Pediatr Emerg Care 2014;30(1):43–6.

15. Fukushima Y, Ray J, Kraus E, et al. A Review and Proposed Rationale for the use of Ultrasonography as a Diagnostic Modality in the Identification of Bone Stress Injuries. J Ultrasound Med 2018. https://doi.org/10.1002/jum.14588.

16. Banal F, Gandjbakhch F, Foltz V, et al. Sensitivity and specificity of ultrasonography in early diagnosis of metatarsal bone stress fractures: a pilot study of 37 patients. J Rheumatol 2009;36(8):1715–9.

17. Hoffman DF, Adams E, Bianchi S. Ultrasonography of fractures in sports medicine. Br J Sports Med 2015;49(3):152–60.

18. Kwee RM, Kwee TC. Ultrasound for diagnosing radiographically occult scaphoid fracture. Skeletal Radiol 2018. https://doi.org/10.1007/s00256-018-2931-7.

19. Senall JA, Failla JM, Bouffard JA, et al. Ultrasound for the early diagnosis of clinically suspected scaphoid fracture1 1No benefits in any form have been received or will be received by a commercial party related directly or indirectly to the subject of this article. J Hand Surg 2004;29(3):400–5.

20. Christiansen TG, Rude C, Lauridsen KK, et al. Diagnostic value of ultrasound in scaphoid fractures. Injury 1991;22(5):397–9.

21. Oguz AB, Polat O, Eneyli MG, et al. The efficiency of bedside ultrasonography in patients with wrist injury and comparison with other radiological imaging methods: A prospective study. Am J Emerg Med 2017;35(6):855–9.

22. Bouillis J, Lallouet S, Ropars M. Echography-Guided Pinning for Prevention of Iatrogenic Injuries to the Radial Nerve during Fixation of Extra-articular Distal Radius Fracture: An Anatomical Study. J wrist Surg 2017;6(4):336–9.

23. Vosbikian MM, Ketonis C, Huang R, et al. Optimal Positioning for Volar Plate Fixation of a Distal Radius Fracture: Determining the Distal Dorsal Cortical Distance. Orthop Clin North Am 2016;47(1):235–44.

24. Imatani J, Akita K, Yamaguchi K, et al. An anatomical study of the watershed line on the volar, distal aspect of the radius: implications for plate placement and avoidance of tendon ruptures. J Hand Surg Am 2012;37(8):1550–4.

25. Obert L, Loisel F, Gasse N, et al. Distal radius anatomy applied to the treatment of wrist fractures by plate: a review of recent literature. SICOT-J. 2015; 1:14.

26. Gurbuz Y, Kucuk L, Gunay H, et al. Comparison of ultrasound and dorsal horizon radiographic view for the detection of dorsal screw penetration. Acta Orthop Traumatol Turc 2017;51(6):448–50.

27. Vernet P, Durry A, Nicolau X, et al. Detection of penetration of the dorsal cortex by epiphyseal screws of distal radius volar plates: Anatomical study comparing ultrasound and fluoroscopy. Orthop Traumatol Surg Res 2017;103(6):911–3.

Ultrasound Elastography for Hand Soft Tissue Assessment

Hugo Giambini, PhD[a],*, Kai-Nan An, PhD[b]

KEYWORDS

- Elastography • Muscle • Tendon • Nerve • Surgery • Injury • Hand

KEY POINTS

- Elastography estimates of tissue properties are valuable measurements for clinical evaluations.
- Elastography techniques allow for passive and active tissue evaluations at various joint positions.
- Shear-wave elastography has several advantages over other elastography imaging techniques.
- Median nerve and tendon properties estimates can be used for the evaluation of carpal tunnel syndrome and carpal tunnel pressure.
- Muscle properties estimates can be used for the evaluation of stroke, spasticity, and/or other pathological conditions.

INTRODUCTION

Abnormal tissue mechanical properties usually characterize diseased or injured tissues. Evaluation of tissue structure and mechanical properties, passive and active tissue, and joint function is of utmost importance in the clinical setting to differentiate healthy subjects from those presenting with a pathology. In 1991, Dr. Jonathan Ophir introduced the concept of ultrasound elastography to measure tissue properties.[1] Elastography has been used for diagnosis in the liver,[2] breast,[3] and other homogeneous tissues. It is until recently that the technique has been implemented in vitro and in vivo in other tissues such as muscle, tendons, and ligaments.

Surgical and rehabilitation objectives, strategies, and procedures are based on the current condition of the tissue and are aimed at improving or changing their properties and/or function. Ultrasound elastography has the potential to aid in this process due to several advantages of the technique including noninvasive imaging, quantitative analysis, real-time evaluations, and the ability to obtain passive and active outcomes. These advantages allow for the evaluation and monitoring of surgical and therapeutic interventions over time and facilitate decision-making directed toward improvement in treatment outcomes. This review article presents a brief description of the theory and fundamentals behind elastography techniques and outlines research and clinical studies in nerves, muscles, tendons, and ligaments of the arm and hands.

PRINCIPLES OF ULTRASOUND ELASTOGRAPHY TECHNIQUES

Elastography techniques aim to describe tissue properties, usually represented by the stiffness of the material, by producing and measuring tissue deformation. The imaging-based stiffness is characterized by the modulus of elasticity (Young's modulus; Pa, Pascal), defined as follows:

$$E = \sigma/\varepsilon \quad (1)$$

where σ is the stress (Pa) and ε is the strain (unitless). Strain is a measurement of the change in

a Department of Biomedical Engineering and Chemical Engineering, University of Texas at San Antonio, College of Engineering and Integrated Design, One UTSA Circle, San Antonio, TX 78249, USA; b Mayo Clinic College of Medicine, 200 First Street, S.W, Rochester, MN 55905, USA
* Corresponding author.
E-mail address: hugo.giambini@utsa.edu

Hand Clin 38 (2022) 119–128
https://doi.org/10.1016/j.hcl.2021.08.013

length, or deformation, of the tissue with an applied load divided by the initial length of the tissue. Various elastography techniques induce and measure tissue deformation differently, and it is based on this difference that the authors describe the techniques.

Quasi-Static Elastography: Strain Elastography

Ultrasound strain elastography measures the strain by estimating the axial deformation of tissue with an externally applied force. Briefly, the operator uses the ultrasound probe to exert a small force (stress) on the subject's body surface, generating a small deformation (strain) of the tissue. Tissue strain, displayed as an elastogram, is then estimated by comparing the deformation of the tissue before and after the application of force. Although theoretically, and based on Equation (1), it is possible to calculate the Young's modulus of the tissue, the stress applied by compressing and decompressing the tissue is unknown, preventing its calculation. Although manual compression using this technique can work well for superficial organs and tissues, its use is challenging when assessing deeper tissues.

Stiffer tissues will deform little with an applied stress compared with larger deformations observed in softer, less stiff, tissues. The qualitative elastograms represented with gray or color scales and describing tissue strain are based on the change of radio frequency signals before and after compression.[4] The qualitative color representation of the elastograms vary depending on the ultrasound equipment and manufacturer.[4] Although elastograms describe qualitative tissue strains, there are several semiquantitative approaches that can be implemented in superficial tissues to obtain a strain ratio (**Fig. 1**).[4,5] One method calculates the average strain from a reference material placed atop the tissue and with known properties, then divides this value with the calculated strain from a deeper tissue.[6] Another method implements a similar approach but uses a superficial tissue (usually subcutaneous fat) to evaluate the properties of a deeper healthy or diseased tissue. Although these semiquantitative approaches provide additional information from tissues, they do not necessarily estimate the intrinsic properties of tissues (ie, modulus/stiffness). In addition, they present inherent limitations associated to operator compression variability and inability to measure superficial tissues due to a lack or very thin subcutaneous fat between the skin and tissue of interest, preventing tissue deformation and generating artifacts.[4,7]

Shear-Wave Elastography

Shear-wave elastography (SWE) uses the shear waves generated in the tissue to quantitatively estimate tissue stiffness (**Fig. 2**). Although shear waves can be generated using external vibrators (transient elastography), the authors focus on the methodology generating shear waves via ultrasound. In 2004, Bercoff and colleagues introduced the concept of supersonic shear imaging (SSI) for the evaluation of tissue elasticity.[8] SSI uses acoustic radiation force to generate low-frequency and higher amplitude shear waves in tissues that radiate transverse to the initial radiation force direction. Briefly, ultrasound push beams are focused at different depths, creating a shear source that moves at a supersonic speed creating quasiplane shear waves. Shear waves will constructively interact and interfere with each other along a cone, creating 2 opposing shear-wave fronts. The resulting transient shear waves are then imaged with the same ultrasound probe at an ultrafast frame rate to obtain local tissue velocities. Assuming a constant density (ρ) of tissue (1000 kg/m^3) tissue shear modulus is calculated as follows (Equation 2)[8]:

$$\mu = \rho c^2 \tag{2}$$

where μ is the shear modulus, ρ is the density of the tissue, and c is the shear wave speed. Assuming linear, homogenous, and isotropic medium, the Young's modulus, as surrogate for tissue stiffness, can then be estimated from the shear-wave speed ($E \sim 3\mu$).[8] Finally, SSI will display quantitative images outcomes superimposed on regular B-mode images.

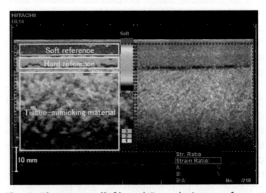

Fig. 1. Elastogram (*left*) and B-mode images from a tissue-mimicking material. The elastogram shows the soft and hard reference materials with a color-coded scale (from red/soft to blue/hard) used to calculate the strain ratio. (*From* Chino K, Akagi R, Dohi M, et al. Reliability and validity of quantifying absolute muscle hardness using ultrasound elastography. PLoS One. 2012;7(9):e45764.Pubmed Partial Page; distributed under the terms of the Creative Commons Attribution License.)

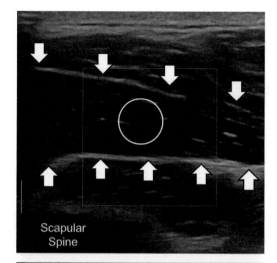

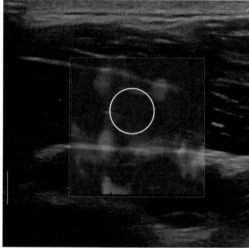

Scapular
Spine

Fig. 2. B-mode (*top*) and elastogram (*bottom*) images using shear-wave elastography. In vivo images from the infraspinatus muscle of the shoulder from a healthy female volunteer. White arrows indicate fascia enclosing the muscle fibers of the muscle.

There are several advantages from using SSI in imaging tissues. These benefits include real-time measurements of tissue stiffness, excellent reproducibility, and acquiring data from tissues or joint positions that would limit the use of external vibrators (such as the case of transient elastography). Although operator dependency is largely limited with this technique, tissue compression with the ultrasound probe can increase tissue stiffness values so care should be taken to impose minimal pressure while obtaining the measurements. On the other hand, there are some limitations to this technique. Based on the fact that this technique assumes isotropy of tissues, anisotropic tissues such as muscles require specific techniques for

acquiring measurements. Although anisotropic properties can be estimated from muscles, the user needs to adapt the imaging process by tilting the probe so that this is aligned parallel to the muscle fibers direction.[9]

APPLICATIONS FOR ASSESSING SOFT TISSUES IN THE HAND BEFORE, DURING, AND POSTSURGERIES

Nerve Imaging—Median Nerve for Carpal Tunnel Syndrome

Over the past ~7 years, most basic and clinical research and review studies implementing and discussing ultrasound elastography imaging on nerves have been on the median nerve (MN) for carpal tunnel syndrome (CTS). In 2013, Orman and colleagues reported the first study discussing the feasibility of ultrasound strain elastography in the diagnosis of CTS. The investigators demonstrated that the stiffness of the MN measured at the wrist was based on the amount of strain observed with the US under a given compression. Results showed mean tissue strain to be significantly lower in patients with CTS (0.094 ± 0.045) when compared with control subjects (0.145 ± 0.068).[10] In 2014, Miyamoto and colleagues reported improvements in the diagnosis of CTS by measuring the elasticity of the MN using a similar technique. MN strain ratio, described as the ratio of the acoustic coupler and the MN, was significantly higher in patients with CTS than healthy subjects (**Fig. 3**).[11] In 2014, Kantarci and colleagues reported the first attempt in using quantitative SWE for the assessment of stiffness of the MN based on wave propagation speed at the level of carpal tunnel inlet. The study investigated 37 patients with CTS and 18 healthy controls, finding higher SWE-measured stiffness values in the MN of patients with CTS (66.7 kPa) compared with normal controls (32.0 kPa). A 40.4-kPa cut-off SWE value established from a receiver-operating curve (ROC) revealed a sensitivity, specificity, positive predictive value, negative predictive value, and accuracy in the diagnosis of CTS based on the cross-sectional area of the carpal tunnel inlet and SWE measurements of 93.3%, 88.9%, 93.3%, 88.9%, and 91.7%, respectively.[12] The investigators suggest long-term edema or high carpal tunnel pressure to lead to the observed increase in MN stiffness. In 2016, Miyamoto and colleagues summarized and discussed in a mini-review the principles, advantages, and disadvantages of compression elastography, or static strain elastography, and SWE in the setting of CTS.[13]

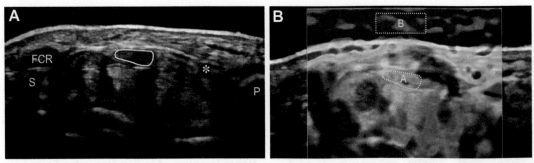

Fig. 3. Transverse images in a 57-year-old healthy female volunteer. (*a*) Conventional B-mode US image shows the MN CSA corresponding to the circle with an area of 8 mm². * = ulnar artery, FCR = flexor carpi radialis, P = pisiform bone, S = scaphoid bone. (*b*) Sonoelastographic image obtained at same level as (*a*). The color represents the elasticity of the tissue within the region of interest, whose scale ranged from red for components with the greatest strain (softest components) to blue for those with no strain (hardest components). The strain ratio of the AC (*B*) to the MN (*A*) was 2.9. AC, acoustic coupler; CSA, cross-sectional area. (*From* Miyamoto H, Halpern E J, Kastlunger M, et al. Carpal Tunnel Syndrome: Diagnosis by Means of Median Nerve Elasticity—Improved Diagnostic Accuracy of US with Sonoelastograph. Radiology 2014; 270:481-486; with permission.)

In 2017, Greening and Dilley reported movement-evoked changes in MN shear-wave velocities measurements from healthy subjects, showing an increase in stiffness with an increase in nerve stretch. Stretching of the nerve may alter its structural morphology and tension, leading to an alteration of stiffness and wave propagation speed. Changes in nerve stiffness associated with movements that lengthen the nerve path have not been examined in detail but may be important in understanding movement-evoked pain in patients with a variety of different musculoskeletal conditions.[14] Paluch and colleagues investigated SWE-measured stiffness on 87 patients with CTS and on 34 control subjects. In order to reduce the variation of absolute SWE-measured stiffness values from nerve tissue, the investigators obtained measurements at various locations, at the level of the proximal carpal row, and at 2 locations proximally on the forearm. SWE imaging outcomes were then normalized by calculating the wrist to forearm stiffness ratios. Similar to Kantarci and colleagues, nerve stiffness values were higher in patients with CTS than normal controls. However, these measurements were much higher than those previously reported, and the cut-off SWE value proposed for nerve stiffness was almost twice that of Kantarci and colleagues (79kPa vs 40.4 kPa). For good diagnostic accuracy and as independent measurements from age and weight, based on the ROC analyses differentiating neuropathic and nonneuropathic subjects, the investigators recommended a wrist-to-forearm ratio of 1.48.[15] In 2018, Bedewi and colleagues implemented SWE on the MN using the same approach as Paluch and colleagues. The variability of outcomes and absolute values for a healthy control group were smaller than those reported by Paluch and colleagues and Kantarci and colleagues. The investigators state several factors affecting the absolute values for tissue stiffness, including anthropometric features, age, sex, ethnicity, equipment, and the location and plane of imaging, suggesting for each laboratory to acquire normal measurements values.[16]

Zhang and colleagues investigated shear-wave velocities in the MN on 49 patients with CTS and 12 healthy volunteers reporting significantly higher outcomes in subjects with CTS (3.857 m/s) compared with controls (2.542 m/s). The investigators suggested a cut-off value of 3.0 m/s with an accuracy rate of 86.4%.[17] Similar to previous studies indicating an increase in SWE values on patients with CTS, Cingoz and colleagues showed higher elasticity values in the MN of 31 patients with CTS (40.8–77.0 kPa) when compared with 9 control subjects (31.0–39.9 kPa). Patients with moderate-to-severe CTS had higher elasticity values (64.0–95.5 kPa) compared with patients with mild CTS (32.5–59.5 kPa).[18] SWE-measured stiffness from patients with CTS and healthy subjects from this group are in the same range as those reported by Kantarci and colleagues.[12] Reliability and feasibility analyses of SWE in the MN and bilateral differences outcomes from 40 healthy subjects showed excellent interobserver and intraobserver agreement (0.852–0.930), with no differences between bilateral forearm measurements.[19] It is important to note that mean values (absolute SWE outcomes) were statistically different at different body sites, that is, if measurements were obtained at the wrist or forearm. Similar to previous studies, SWE-measured stiffness, or wave velocities, increased with stretch of the MN as the wrist was placed in an extended posture.

Evaluation of the MN using elastography has also been performed on other pathologies subjects. In 2019, He and colleagues implemented SWE to evaluate the stiffness of the MN in 40 subjects with diabetic peripheral neuropathy (DPN), 40 subjects with diabetes mellitus (DM), and 40 healthy subjects. MN stiffness was significantly higher in patients with DPN compared with healthy volunteers and patients with DM, showing the feasibility of SWE for assisting in the diagnosis of DPN.[20] During the same year, a publication by Lin and colleagues reported a comprehensive review and meta-analysis of compression strain-type and SWE techniques in the assessment of MN in CTS.[21] Pubmed and Embase databases were used to include the earliest record upto April 2019, comprising 17 studies, evaluating 1401 wrists. The primary search evaluation and outcome was a comparison of MN elasticity between patients with CTS and those without CTS. Comparisons were performed by quantifying the standard mean difference (SMD), derived from the mean difference of elasticity between the groups and divided by the pooled standard deviations, and its 95% confidence interval. MN was considered stiffer in the subjects with CTS compared with controls when the SMD of tissue strain was negative, or that of strain ratio, and the shear-wave velocity was positive. Conclusive remarks from the analyses showed consistent higher stiffness values in patients with CTS compared with healthy subjects regardless of the ultrasound elastography mode being implemented (tissue strain, strain ratio, shear modulus, and shear-wave velocity) and emphasized ultrasound elastography as a potential imaging tool in differentiating CTS of various severities.

Concluding the authors' review of studies addressing MN and CTS, in 2019, Zakrzewski and colleagues reported a comprehensive review of ultrasound elastography in the evaluation of peripheral neuropathies, including CTS and other entrapment neuropathies, and DPN and peripheral neuropathy associated with other systemic diseases.[22] Finally, in 2020, Yoshii and colleagues used strain elastography (compression elastography) to estimate the elasticity of the MN based on the applied pressure and strain ratio.[23,24] Similar to previous research, the investigators found a significant increase in MN strain, suggesting the pressure-strain ratio as a reliable marker reflecting clinical recovery and tissue properties after surgery.

Muscle Imaging—Intrinsic Muscle Contracture and Stroke Spastic Contracture

In 2010, Gennisson and colleagues performed a comprehensive assessment of the viscoelastic properties of the biceps using SWE, documenting factors affecting the measurements and proposing potential clinical applications.[25] Shear modulus and shear viscosity were quantitatively assessed assuming the viscoelastic Voigt's model. In 2013, Eby and colleagues validated the measurements of muscle stiffness obtained using SWE directly from mechanical testing evaluations.[9] SWE measurements were obtained by manipulating the alignment of the ultrasound transducer with respect to the long axis of the muscle fibers, demonstrating that a simple relation based on isotropic material assumptions was not appropriate. In 2014, Brandenburg and colleagues reviewed ultrasound elastography technologies applied in the assessment of muscles during rehabilitation applications.[26] Strain elastography, acoustic radiation force impulse, transient elastography, and supersonic shear imaging techniques were discussed, and potential applications with future directions were identified. In 2015, Koo and Hug reported on the assessment of muscle stiffness using SWE during passive stretching.[27] Variables affecting the increase in SWE-measured stiffness during stretching were discussed based on a widely accepted Hill-type passive force-length relationship model. The model, validated against ex vivo animal data previously reported by the same group,[28] suggested that *"resting shear modulus of a slack muscle is a function of specific tension and parameters that govern the normalized passive muscle force–length relationship as well as the degree of muscle anisotropy."* A take home message from the investigators stated that *"while the slope of the linear resting shear modulus vs. passive force relationship was primarily related to the anatomic cross-section of the muscle (ie,: the smaller the muscle cross-sectional area, the larger the increase in shear modulus to result in the same passive muscle force), it was also governed by the normalized passive muscle force–length relationship and the degree of muscle anisotropy."*

In 2015, Lee and colleagues implemented SWE to assess the material properties in spastic-paretic muscles (biceps brachii) and contralateral muscles from stroke survivors (**Fig. 4**).[29] SWE-measured stiffness was altered in stroke-impaired muscles at rest, indicating the potential for this technique in the evaluation of muscles in patients with stroke and during clinical examinations. In 2016, Eby and colleagues quantified passive stiffness, or shear

Non-paretic   Paretic

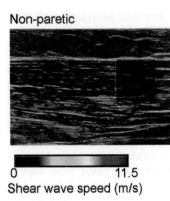
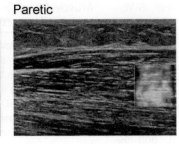

0   11.5
Shear wave speed (m/s)

Fig. 4. Shear-wave (SW) ultrasound elastography images of the nonparetic and paretic biceps brachii muscles of a representative subject. The squares represent the region of interest from which SW speed was measured. In these images, the nonparetic muscle has a mean SW speed of 2.5 m/s, whereas the paretic muscle has a mean SW speed of 4.7 m/s. (*Reprinted from* Clinical Biomechanics, Volume 30, Issue 3, Sabrina S.M. Lee, Sam Spear, William Z. Rymer, Quantifying changes in material properties of stroke-impaired muscle, Pages 269-275, March 2015, with permission from Elsevier.)

modulus, using SWE of the biceps brachii throughout adulthood in flexed and extended elbow positions, showing increased stiffness values with increasing age and higher outcomes in women compared with men.[30] Eby and colleagues also implemented SWE in the biceps brachii muscle of subjects with stroke during passive elbow extension.[31] Approximately half of the subjects with stroke showed an increase in joint torque during elbow extension, as measured with a dynamometer, coupled with a comparable increase in muscle SWE-measured stiffness. Along with joint stiffness measurements, the study delineated the relative contributions of muscle spasticity and joint contracture. In 2017, Wu and colleagues evaluated the stiffness of biceps brachii muscles at 90° and 0° elbow flexion in 31 patients who had recent strokes and on 21 control subjects.[32] The study showed high shear-wave velocities to be associated with high spasticity and poor function of the poststroke upper limb. In 2019, Watanabe and colleagues investigated the stiffness of the first dorsal interosseous and lumbrical muscles in the hand using SWE as a function of finger joint position and wrist rotation.[33] The purpose of the study was to develop a method for assessing the stiffness of the intrinsic muscles of the hand in the evaluation or treatment of muscle contracture. Finally, in 2020, Lehoux and colleagues published a comprehensive literature review of SWE as a potential tool to characterize spastic muscles in stroke survivors.[34]

Tendon Imaging—Tendon Pathology, Tension During Transfer, Tendon as Gauge for Estimation of Carpal Tunnel Pressure

In 2014, DeWall and colleagues implemented SWE to assess wave propagation and regional tendon properties with various degree of lacerations

(**Fig. 5**).[35] The investigators recognized the limitation in the application of the technique to tendons due to the fast shear-wave propagations in the very stiff tendons and the constraint in data acquisition, especially with stretched tissue. Nevertheless, they observed changes in stiffness (ie, speed) at the vicinity, before and after, of the tendon laceration, showing the potential of the technique in the evaluation of tendon injuries. Expanding on the application of elastography to tendons, in 2014, Ooi and colleagues reviewed the implementation and limitations of axial-strain sonoelastography and SWE in the assessment of tendon injuries.[36] In general, although extensive studies were included using axial-strain compression elastography for assessing tendon properties, unfortunately, the technique showed significant barriers such as operator dependency and limited reproducibility. On the other hand, although SWE can overcome some of these limitations, few studies were reported in the review due to its limited implementation in tendons. In 2016, Roskoff and colleagues correlated the force applied to a tendon with shear-wave velocity outcomes from 2 different elastography equipments.[37] Shear-wave velocities depend highly on the mechanical forces in the tendon tissue, emphasizing reproducibility and reliability issues with applied loads. However, reproducible and comparable measurements from different ultrasound systems were addressed by controlling the applied load.

In 2016, Yeh and colleagues reported a comprehensive study using SWE to obtain properties of tendon tissue damaged by collagenase digestion.[38] Results from the study showed an increase in Young's modulus and shear modulus, estimated from mechanical testing and elastography, respectively, with increasing preloads applied to the tendon. Shear modulus outcomes were lower in collagenase-treated tendons. Although there

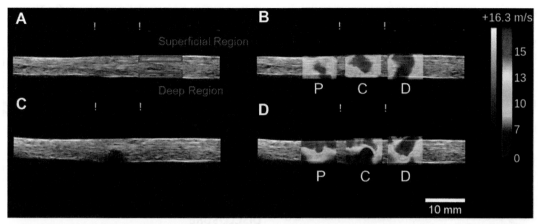

Fig. 5. Comparison of tendon before (*A, B*) and after tearing to 75% (*C, D*) of tendon thickness. Shear-wave speed was estimated in regions of interest left of (*L*), centered on (*C*) and right of (*R*) the tear. The deep-to-superficial ratio was measured using the top and bottom quarters of each ROI, as shown in the right ROI in (*A*). In all cases, the area within the cut was excluded. (*Reprinted from* Ultrasound in Medicine & Biology, Volume 40, Issue 1, Ryan J. DeWall, Jingfeng Jiang, John J. Wilson, Kenneth S.Lee, Visualizing Tendon Elasticity in an ex Vivo Partial Tear Model, Pages 158-167, January 2014, with permission from Elsevier.)

can be bias in SWE-measured modulus associated with the dispersion of shear waves in tendons and their wavelengths being greater than the tendon thickness, SWE still detected significant differences between normal and collagenase-damaged tendon properties. In 2017, Lamouille and colleagues reported the assessment of in vivo muscle tension during transfer of the extensor indicis proprius to the extensor pollicis longus.[39] SWE measurements were obtained at different stages of surgery including at rest, during active extension, and after tendon transfer at rest. The investigators showed differences in SWE-measured stiffness at the various stages of the tendon transfer procedure, demonstrating such measurements to be beneficial with potential of improving therapeutic treatments of tendon transfers. In 2017, Turkay and colleagues evaluated the feasibility of SWE in detecting degenerative tendons associated with tenosynovitis.[40] The group assessed extensor compartment tendons and its alterations with tenosynovitis in 40 healthy volunteers and 40 de Quervain patients. The median SWE value of the de Quervain patient group was lower by ~2.5-fold compared with the healthy group (29 kPa vs 72 kPa), showing statistically significant differences. ROC analyses led to a 40.5 kPa SWE cut-off value for the diagnosis of de Quervain tenosynovitis with 95% specificity and 85% sensitivity.

In 2017, Domenichini and colleagues presented an excellent review of elastography techniques, including quasi-static elastography, acoustic radiation force imaging, and SWE, for assessing various tendons pathologies.[7] Theoretical considerations, fundamentals, and challenges associated to multiple tendons (achilles, patellar, rotator cuff, and so forth) were included in the review. In 2018, Martin and colleagues demonstrated the potential for evaluating noninvasive in vivo tendon loads based on shear-wave propagation, using SWE or instrumented tapping and accelerometers, during isometric exertions, walking, and running.[41] In addition to the MN, Lee and colleagues assessed the stiffness of the flexor digitorum profundus and flexor digitorum superficialis tendons and of the transverse carpal ligament using acoustic radiation force impulse elastography. Evaluations of these structures were performed at various wrist and finger join postures.[42] In 2019, Sendur and colleagues implemented SWE to measure the stiffness of the common extensor tendon known to be associated with lateral epicondylopathy or tennis elbow.[43] The imaging process was reproducible, suggesting that data from healthy volunteers could be used for comparison in the evaluation of pathologic subjects. In 2020, Hsiao and colleagues described the implementation of high-frequency ultrasound–SWE to characterize the extensor digitorum communis tendon.[44] The process was able to measure wave speeds upto 135 m/s, correlating with tendon forces upto 50% of maximum voluntary contraction. Finally, flexor tendon properties have been evaluated to gauge carpal tunnel pressure showing a linear relationship between the change in tendon rigidity, as measured using SWE, and the applied compressive pressure.[45–48] Rigidity measurements from a single tendon region, inside and outside the tunnel, were able to estimate pressure outcomes.

FUTURE DEVELOPMENT

Ultrasound elastography allows for quantitative measurements of tissue properties for diagnosis, pretreatment planning, and posttreatment evaluations. Elastography techniques are valuable in detecting changes in tissue properties that occur due to injury, disease, and/or treatments. In the setting of CTS, elastography can be implemented to evaluate nerve and tendon stiffness and changes in stiffness outcomes with increase pressures. Soft tissue injuries in the hand, including ligaments, the triangular fibrocartilage complex, or skin and subcutaneous changes in properties, such as in Dupuytren's contracture, are other potential applications for elastography techniques to improve the diagnosis and interpretation of clinical outcomes. Similarly, pretreatment planning can be improved by considering elastography evaluations in the process, as is the case of stiffness evaluations from candidate muscles and tendons for a tendon transfer procedure.

Although there exists significant potential in the application of elastography in the clinic for diagnosis (such as muscle contracture, neuropathies, tendon repairs), surgical assistance (such as muscle and tendon tension adjustment in tendon transfers), and rehabilitation (such as spastic muscle evaluations from stroke), there are still questions to be answered and some work left to be done to improve the process and further understand the potential and limitations in measurements. Absolute SWE outcomes from passive conditions have been shown to differ from active measurements. Should the focus in measurements be on passive or active muscle conditions? Is a specific joint position optimum for understanding tissue properties, function, or disease? Does sex and age affect outcomes? Do individual muscle compartments have similar roles in joint and muscle function? Answers to some of these questions have been attempted and significant improvements have been made toward validating the technique and standardizing values. As real-time, noninvasive, and quantitative measurements of tissue stiffness continue to be collected, big-data emerges as a potential field where outcome measurements can be analyzed and information can be extracted and compared with a population of normative and pathologic subjects.

CLINICS CARE POINTS

- Elastography can be implemented in the clinic to aid diagnosis, treatment, and rehabilitation of various conditions.
- Elastography can be used to asses properties of muscles, nerves, and ligaments.
- Normalized imaging approaches and measurements is required for an appropriate clinical application.

DISCLOSURE

This study was supported by the University of Texas at San Antonio.

REFERENCES

1. Ophir J, Cespedes I, Ponnekanti H, et al. Elastography: a quantitative method for imaging the elasticity of biological tissues. Ultrason Imaging 1991;13(2):111–34.
2. Barr RG. Shear wave liver elastography. Abdom Radiol (N Y) 2018;43(4):800–7.
3. Zhu QL, Jiang YX, Liu JB, et al. Real-time ultrasound elastography: its potential role in assessment of breast lesions. Ultrasound Med Biol 2008;34(8):1232–8.
4. Carlsen JF, Ewertsen C, Lonn L, et al. Strain elastography ultrasound: an overview with emphasis on breast cancer diagnosis. Diagnostics (Basel) 2013;3(1):117–25.
5. Franchi-Abella S, Elie C, Correas JM. Ultrasound elastography: advantages, limitations and artefacts of the different techniques from a study on a phantom. Diagn Interv Imaging 2013;94(5):497–501.
6. Chino K, Akagi R, Dohi M, et al. Reliability and validity of quantifying absolute muscle hardness using ultrasound elastography. PLoS One 2012;7(9):e45764.
7. Domenichini R, Pialat JB, Podda A, et al. Ultrasound elastography in tendon pathology: state of the art. Skeletal Radiol 2017;46(12):1643–55.
8. Bercoff J, Tanter M, Fink M. Supersonic shear imaging: a new technique for soft tissue elasticity mapping. IEEE Trans Ultrason Ferroelectr Freq Control 2004;51(4):396–409.
9. Eby SF, Song P, Chen S, et al. Validation of shear wave elastography in skeletal muscle. J Biomech 2013;46(14):2381–7.
10. Orman G, Ozben S, Huseyinoglu N, et al. Ultrasound elastographic evaluation in the diagnosis of carpal tunnel syndrome: initial findings. Ultrasound Med Biol 2013;39(7):1184–9.

11. Miyamoto H, Halpern EJ, Kastlunger M, et al. Carpal tunnel syndrome: diagnosis by means of median nerve elasticity–improved diagnostic accuracy of US with sonoelastography. Radiology 2014;270(2):481–6.

12. Kantarci F, Ustabasioglu FE, Delil S, et al. Median nerve stiffness measurement by shear wave elastography: a potential sonographic method in the diagnosis of carpal tunnel syndrome. Eur Radiol 2014;24(2):434–40.

13. Miyamoto H, Morizaki Y, Kashiyama T, et al. Grey-scale sonography and sonoelastography for diagnosing carpal tunnel syndrome. World J Radiol 2016;8(3):281–7.

14. Greening J, Dilley A. Posture-induced changes in peripheral nerve stiffness measured by ultrasound shear-wave elastography. Muscle Nerve 2017;55(2):213–22.

15. Paluch L, Pietruski P, Walecki J, et al. Wrist to forearm ratio as a median nerve shear wave elastography test in carpal tunnel syndrome diagnosis. J Plast Reconstr Aesthet Surg 2018;71(8):1146–52.

16. Bedewi MA, Coraci D, Ruggeri F, et al. Shear wave elastography of median nerve at wrist and forearm. Heterogeneity of normative values. J Plast Reconstr Aesthet Surg 2019;72(1):137–71.

17. Zhang C, Li M, Jiang J, et al. Diagnostic value of virtual touch tissue imaging quantification for evaluating median nerve stiffness in carpal tunnel syndrome. J Ultrasound Med 2017;36(9):1783–91.

18. Cingoz M, Kandemirli SG, Alis DC, et al. Evaluation of median nerve by shear wave elastography and diffusion tensor imaging in carpal tunnel syndrome. Eur J Radiol 2018;101:59–64.

19. Zhu B, Yan F, He Y, et al. Evaluation of the healthy median nerve elasticity: Feasibility and reliability of shear wave elastography. Medicine (Baltimore) 2018;97(43):e12956.

20. He Y, Xiang X, Zhu BH, et al. Shear wave elastography evaluation of the median and tibial nerve in diabetic peripheral neuropathy. Quant Imaging Med Surg 2019;9(2):273–82.

21. Lin CP, Chen IJ, Chang KV, et al. Utility of ultrasound elastography in evaluation of carpal tunnel syndrome: a systematic review and meta-analysis. Ultrasound Med Biol 2019;45(11):2855–65.

22. Zakrzewski J, Zakrzewska K, Pluta K, et al. Ultrasound elastography in the evaluation of peripheral neuropathies: a systematic review of the literature. Pol J Radiol 2019;84:e581–91.

23. Yoshii Y, Tung WL, Ishii T. Measurement of median nerve strain and applied pressure for the diagnosis of carpal tunnel syndrome. Ultrasound Med Biol 2017;43(6):1205–9.

24. Yoshii Y, Tung WL, Yuine H, et al. Postoperative diagnostic potentials of median nerve strain and applied pressure measurement after carpal tunnel release. BMC Musculoskelet Disord 2020;21(1):22.

25. Gennisson JL, Deffieux T, Mace E, et al. Viscoelastic and anisotropic mechanical properties of in vivo muscle tissue assessed by supersonic shear imaging. Ultrasound Med Biol 2010;36(5):789–801.

26. Brandenburg JE, Eby SF, Song P, et al. Ultrasound elastography: the new frontier in direct measurement of muscle stiffness. Arch Phys Med Rehabil 2014;95(11):2207–19.

27. Koo TK, Hug F. Factors that influence muscle shear modulus during passive stretch. J Biomech 2015;48(12):3539–42.

28. Koo TK, Guo JY, Cohen JH, et al. Relationship between shear elastic modulus and passive muscle force: an ex-vivo study. J Biomech 2013;46(12):2053–9.

29. Lee SS, Spear S, Rymer WZ. Quantifying changes in material properties of stroke-impaired muscle. Clin Biomech (Bristol, Avon) 2015;30(3):269–75.

30. Eby SF, Cloud BA, Brandenburg JE, et al. Shear wave elastography of passive skeletal muscle stiffness: influences of sex and age throughout adulthood. Clin Biomech (Bristol, Avon) 2015;30(1):22–7.

31. Eby S, Zhao H, Song P, et al. Quantitative evaluation of passive muscle stiffness in chronic stroke. Am J Phys Med Rehabil 2016;95(12):899–910.

32. Wu CH, Ho YC, Hsiao MY, et al. Evaluation of post-stroke spastic muscle stiffness using shear wave ultrasound elastography. Ultrasound Med Biol 2017;43(6):1105–11.

33. Watanabe Y, Iba K, Taniguchi K, et al. Assessment of the passive tension of the first dorsal interosseous and first lumbrical muscles using shear wave elastography. J Hand Surg Am 2019;44(12):1092.e1–18.

34. Lehoux MC, Sobczak S, Cloutier F, et al. Shear wave elastography potential to characterize spastic muscles in stroke survivors: literature review. Clin Biomech (Bristol, Avon) 2020;72:84–93.

35. Dewall RJ, Jiang J, Wilson JJ, et al. Visualizing tendon elasticity in an ex vivo partial tear model. Ultrasound Med Biol 2014;40(1):158–67.

36. Ooi CC, Malliaras P, Schneider ME, et al. "Soft, hard, or just right?" Applications and limitations of axial-strain sonoelastography and shear-wave elastography in the assessment of tendon injuries. Skeletal Radiol 2014;43(1):1–12.

37. Rosskopf AB, Bachmann E, Snedeker JG, et al. Comparison of shear wave velocity measurements assessed with two different ultrasound systems in an ex-vivo tendon strain phantom. Skeletal Radiol 2016;45(11):1541–51.

38. Yeh CL, Kuo PL, Gennisson JL, et al. Shear wave measurements for evaluation of tendon diseases. IEEE Trans Ultrason Ferroelectr Freq Control 2016;63(11):1906–21.

39. Lamouille J, Muller C, Aubry S, et al. Extensor indicis proprius tendon transfer using shear wave elastography. Hand Surg Rehabil 2017;36(3):173–80.

40. Turkay R, Inci E, Aydeniz B, et al. Shear wave elastography findings of de Quervain tenosynovitis. Eur J Radiol 2017;95:192–6.

41. Martin JA, Brandon SCE, Keuler EM, et al. Gauging force by tapping tendons. Nat Commun 2018;9(1): 1592.

42. Lee S, Kwak J, Lee S, et al. Quantitative stiffness of the median nerve, flexor tendons, and flexor retinaculum in the carpal tunnel measured with acoustic radiation force impulse elastography in various wrist and finger positions. Medicine (Baltimore) 2019; 98(36):e17066.

43. Sendur HN, Cindil E, Cerit M, et al. Interobserver variability and stiffness measurements of normal common extensor tendon in healthy volunteers using shear wave elastography. Skeletal Radiol 2019; 48(1):137–41.

44. Hsiao YY, Yang TH, Chen PY, et al. Characterization of the extensor digitorum communis tendon using high-frequency ultrasound shear wave elastography. Med Phys 2020;47(4):1609–18.

45. Cheng YS, Zhou B, Kubo K, et al. Comparison of two ways of altering carpal tunnel pressure with ultrasound surface wave elastography. J Biomech 2018;74:197–201.

46. Kubo K, Cheng YS, Zhou B, et al. The quantitative evaluation of the relationship between the forces applied to the palm and carpal tunnel pressure. J Biomech 2018;66:170–4.

47. Kubo K, Zhou B, Cheng YS, et al. Ultrasound elastography for carpal tunnel pressure measurement: a cadaveric validation study. J Orthop Res 2018; 36(1):477–83.

48. Wang Y, Qiang B, Zhang X, et al. A non-invasive technique for estimating carpal tunnel pressure by measuring shear wave speed in tendon: a feasibility study. J Biomech 2012;45(16):2927–30.

Moving?

Make sure your subscription moves with you!

To notify us of your new address, find your **Clinics Account Number** (located on your mailing label above your name), and contact customer service at:

Email: journalscustomerservice-usa@elsevier.com

800-654-2452 (subscribers in the U.S. & Canada)
314-447-8871 (subscribers outside of the U.S. & Canada)

Fax number: 314-447-8029

Elsevier Health Sciences Division
Subscription Customer Service
3251 Riverport Lane
Maryland Heights, MO 63043

*To ensure uninterrupted delivery of your subscription, please notify us at least 4 weeks in advance of move.